Y0-BYB-585

Occupational Therapy for People With Eating Dysfunctions

The *Occupational Therapy in Health Care* series,
Florence S. Cromwell, Editor

Occupational Therapy for People With Eating Dysfunctions

Florence S. Cromwell
Editor

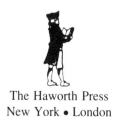

The Haworth Press
New York • London

Occupational Therapy for People With Eating Dysfunctions has also been published as *Occupational Therapy in Health Care,* Volume 3, Number 2, Summer 1986.

The Haworth Press, Inc., 28 East 22 Street, New York, NY 10010-6194
EUROSPAN/Haworth, 3 Henrietta Street, London WC2E 8LU England

Library of Congress Cataloging in Publication Data

Occupational therapy for people with eating dysfunctions.

    "Has also been published as Occupational therapy in health care, volume 3, number
2, summer 1986"—T.p. verso.
    Includes bibliographies.
    1. Appetite disorders—Treatment. 2. Occupational therapy. I. Cromwell, Florence S.
RC552.A72036   1986   617'.43   86-12016
ISBN 0-86656-588-4

Occupational Therapy
for People With Eating Dysfunctions

Occupational Therapy in Health Care
Volume 3, Number 2

CONTENTS

Occupational Therapy for People With Eating Dysfunctions

FROM THE EDITOR'S DESK

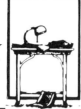

As the professionals most concerned with activities of daily living, we occupational therapists naturally identify with all the tasks and routines associated with daily self-care and self-maintenance as well as with work and leisure. It is not surprising, therefore, to realize that occupational therapists have become *the* specialists in identifying and remediating *eating difficulties* regardless of cause. What could be a more fundamental activity of daily living, and if impaired, more threatening to not only quality of life, but life itself?

Yet, the literature has not comprehensively documented the breadth or depth of the profession's skills and interests in this area of treatment. Yes, there has long been documented the concern with the eating problems encountered by children with cerebral palsy or with mental retardation. Occupational therapists were the originators of much of the adapted equipment used to aid eating when they solved eating difficulties of patients who otherwise would have been 'fed' when weakened or paralyzed by poliomyelitis. Those devices and their successes led naturally to their use in treatment programs for patients with spinal cord quadriplegia, stroke and other neurological conditions. Every age group or disability that presented mechanical problems of getting food to the mouth was not the concern of occupational therapists through the years. Now many of the occupational therapist designed devices are commonplace additions to hospitals, nursing homes and even to the homes of individuals who have learned how handy and helpful a scoop dish or a kni-fork can be.

Then as the profession's skills and knowledge expanded, along

1

with developing neurological and medical science, therapists were called upon to help with the kinds of problems particular to persons with oral motor deficits, behavioral eating problems or swallowing difficulties occurring in populations as diverse as the premature infant to the surgical patient with head and neck cancer to the elder with dementia. Yet all this kind of expertise is only spottily known about. We occupational therapists do well in hiding our skills from view under the breadth of daily living skills we address in today's practice.

While physicians and families may look to nurses or speech therapists as the logical ones to attend to eating, eating difficulties/ oral motor deficits, few of those professional disciplines have either the expertise to assess eating problems in their totality or to carry out daily training routines which sometimes require extraordinary time and patience. While occupational therapists certainly must collaborate with nurses and speech therapists, dietitians and physicians in identifying and planning programs for remediating eating problems, they alone have the undergirding knowledge and philosophy of care that includes ability to address such needs.

When this issue of *OTHC* on the occupational therapist's role in eating programs was conceived, it came as the result of escalating need for expanded knowledge in addressing eating problems being seen among neonates, patients with dramatic structural changes in their eating 'apparatus' as the result of surgery and the growing need for help among the rapidly rising populations of elderly whose competencies in every day living activity may be threatened or impaired. Meal activities, primary socializers for the lone aged person, the nursing home resident, the ill whose capabilities for maintaining independence and life style patterns are compromised by assorted physical, mental and environmental factors. Persons with obvious physical or psychological impediments to eating behaviors continue to be the concern of occupational therapy services.

Thus this issue has taken shape, first from an appeal to readers of the AOTA Newspaper for those interested in sharing with colleagues their eating/feeding program ideas. Over 50 therapists replied. Then as news of the plan for the issue spread, others who were seriously committed to eating programs in their own facilities offered to write of them. As editor my only surprise with the resulting collection is the lack of content regarding eating/feeding programs with some of the most traditional and numerous patient groups occupational therapists see and for whom eating activities may be primary concerns. Those are patients with spinal cord injury, stroke, arthritis, head trauma. Needless to say, the absence of reports of programs with such populations merely indicates to me the certain acceptance of the occupational therapy role in ADL treatment, including eating programs, and the assumption that there is "nothing new to share." Whether the latter is so or not, so be it for now.

In this issue there is richness of both basic and new knowledge about eating activities and deficits, and good examples of how occupational therapists address the needs of such populations. The papers assembled collectively provide a rich resource for clinicians and students alike. Read, discuss and profit from what your colleagues have written. Patients in occupational therapy will certainly be aided by your expanded knowledge.

In the special feature, PRACTICE WATCH, we again share some important ideas for occupational therapists to think about. Given the special values occupational therapists bring to their daily roles, and the high potential for burnout among health professionals who feel the stresses of a changing system, the two papers which make up the feature provide important insights for occupational therapists. Read Madill et al. to see if *your* values match those of your colleagues countrywide and if your practice reflects the implications of those values. Then see how Brollier and her fellow authors look at burnout, the jargon for the condition many in high stress, high productivity jobs feel. Occupational therapists certainly often fit the model of being suspect for burnout. Read to acquire some strategies for prevention for yourself and your fellow staff.

In our second feature, SOMETHING NEW AND USEFUL, Mason and Okkema share information on a simple device which surely will find an acceptance among therapists who work with persons with spinal cord injury. They seek your reaction and response. Our second series of Book Reviews on timely publications concludes the issue.

Volume III of *OTHC* is now at the halfway point. Ahead are two interesting volumes, widely divergent in content. Responding to increasing need for communications technology, the Fall/Winter 1986 issue will address *Computer Applications in Occupational Therapy*. A wide variety of topics is planned to either introduce you to the technology or move you to new applications. Following that, the Spring 1987 issue will look at *Cultural Implications of Treatment*

Planning. Following basic philosophies of the profession which avow interest in total needs of persons served, this series of papers will examine the many ways in which occupational therapists both serve diverse cultures and attend to the culture-specific needs of their patients.

Finally, we continue to invite your suggestions, reactions and responses to the themes and content of *OTHC*. As we are looking ahead to future volumes, we need your input.

Florence S. Cromwell
Editor

Dysphagia in the Adult Population: The Role of Occupational Therapy

Ina Elfant Asher, MS, OTR/L

ABSTRACT. Occupational therapists, traditionally concerned with activities of daily living, are now addressing the problems of eating caused by dysphagia. Adult-onset dysphagia results from either neurological or mechanical, i.e., structural, causes. Following a description of the normal swallowing process, this paper reviews the various disorders that cause dysphagia. General evaluation principles are offered with treatment methods appropriate to the category of disorders. Although specific treatment methods have been used clinically, many remain untested. More recently, a growing number of studies have been published which measure the effectiveness of rehabilitation for dysphagics. Active intervention in the problem of adult-onset dysphagia consists largely of detailed evaluation of oral structures, manipulation of diet, techniques to elicit normal swallowing mechanisms, and assistive devices to compensate for lost structures. In addition, cognitive status, nutrition, posture, and position are addressed in a comprehensive therapy program. The goal of treatment is to promote a safe and nutritional oral diet to the fullest extent possible.

Occupational therapists have always considered the domain of activities of daily living as a primary concern. It is obvious then that occupational therapists should address the problems of self-feeding caused by dysphagia. Until recently, clients with swallowing impairments were treated supportively by the medical profession. That is, if drugs or surgery could not correct the problem, feeding tubes were introduced to maintain the individual's nutritional status. If recovery did not occur spontaneously, the supportive measures were maintained indefinitely.

Ina Elfant Asher, Instructor, Occupational Therapy, Thomas Jefferson University, College of Allied Health Sciences, Philadelphia, PA.

This article appears jointly in *Occupational Therapy for People With Eating Dysfunctions* (The Haworth Press, Inc., 1986) and *Occupational Therapy in Health Care*, Volume 3, Number 2 (Summer 1986).

5

In recent years, health care professionals have begun to explore methods of active intervention in the management of dysphagic clients. These include more detailed evaluation of the oral structures involved in swallowing, manipulation of the diet to promote safer and easier intake of foods, proper positioning, and rehabilitation techniques to stimulate the swallowing structures. Although most of these procedures were developed through clinical trial, their effectiveness has remained largely untested. The past few years, however, have seen an increase of studies measuring the effect of rehabilitation on dysphagia.

First, an overview of the normal swallowing process and the neurologic and mechanical disorders of swallowing will be presented. Next, the general principles of evaluation as well as treatment methods utilized for medical and surgical dysphagic adults will be discussed. The reader is referred to the bibliography for further background on the swallowing mechanisms, pathology and details of the measures described.

NORMAL SWALLOWING

Deglutition is the normal consumption of solids and liquids, and involves a complex interaction of voluntary and reflex activity. It consists of formulation of a bolus in the mouth, propelling it into the pharynx while preventing any particles from entering the nasopharynx or larynx, and transit of residual material through the pharnyngoesophageal tract. Three stages are involved in the swallowing process: the oral, pharnyngeal, and esophageal stages (Figure 1). The following description is condensed from the works of Donner and of Larsen.[1,2] The reader is also referred to the texts by Roueche and by Groher, the latter containing detailed chapters on the physiology and pathology of swallowing.[3,4]

In the oral stage, the food materials placed in the mouth are transported to the pharynx. This is primarily a voluntary process. The oral cavity extends from the lips posteriorly to the pharynx, bordered superiorly by the hard and soft palate and containing the teeth, gums, and tongue. During the oral stage, the bolus is prepared for swallowing by salivation and chewing. The tongue maneuvers it into position: as the tongue tip rises to compress the bolus against the hard palate, the posterior tongue and buccal muscles work the

Figure 1

The Normal Swallow
(reprinted from Schultz[5] with
permission from publisher and
author)

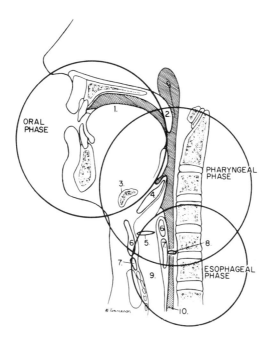

The normal swallow involves three separate
stages that are interdependent and highly coordinated:
(1) tongue, (2) soft palate, (3) hyoid bone, (4) epiglottis,
(5) vocal folds, (6) thyroid cartilage, (7) cricoid cartilage,
(8) pharyngoesophageal sphincter, (9) trachea, and
(10) esophagus.

bolus back toward the pharynx. Tongue retraction and elevation
push the bolus into the upper pharynx while respiration is reflex-
ively inhibited. Sensory input of the oral cavity helps to initiate
swallowing;[6] when food is placed on the tongue, sensory information from the face and oral cavity is transmitted to the brain stem via
cranial nerves, V, VII, IX, X, and XII. (See Figure 2.)

AFFERENT CONTROLS INVOLVED IN SWALLOWING

General sensation, anterior two-thirds of tongue	·Lingual nerve, trigeminal (V)
Taste, anterior two-thirds tongue	Chorda tympani, facial (VII)
Taste and general sensation, posterior one-third of the tongue	Glossopharyngeal (IX)
Mucosa of vallecula Primary afferent	Internal branch of SLN (vagus) Glossopharyngeal (IX)
Secondary afferent Tonsils, pharynx, soft palate	Pharyngeal branch of vagus (X) Glossopharyngeal (IX)
Pharynx, larynx, viscera	Vagus (X)

EFFERENT CONTROLS INVOLVED IN SWALLOWING

Oral

Masticatory, buccinator, floor of mouth	Trigeminal (V)
Lip sphincter	Facial (VII)
Tongue	Hypoglossal (XII)

Pharyngeal

Constrictors and stylopharyngeus	Glossopharyngeal (IX)
Palate, pharynx, larynx	Vagus (X)
Tongue	Hypoglossal (XII)

Esophageal

Esophagus	Vagus (X)

Figure 2: Cranial nerve regulation of oral and facial functions (reprinted from Groher with permission from the publisher and editor).

The pharyngeal stage begins as the bolus is forced into the pharynx. The pharynx is the common passageway for food heading into the esophagus and for air passing into the larynx and pharynx. In this predominantly reflexive phase involving cranial nerves IX, X, and XII, several protective mechanisms guard against aspiration. As the bolus reaches the faucial arches, the swallowing reflex is triggered. This reflex elevates the larynx, bringing the epiglottis to the base of the tongue to block the airway. Pharyngeal muscle peristalsis moves the bolus towards the esophagus, and the vocal cords close off the trachea to protect the airway as well. The cricopharyngeal sphincter muscle is situated at the entrance to the upper esophagus. At the peak of pharyngeal muscle contraction, the tonic contraction of the cricopharyngeus is momentarily inhibited. This relaxation of the sphincter allows the food to pass into the esophagus, completing the pharyngeal phase.

Following relaxation of the cricopharyngeal sphincter muscle, the esophageal phase commences. The bolus passes into the esophagus and is carried to the stomach by peristalsis and gravity, primarily involving cranial nerve X. By this phase, respiration has resumed and the larynx has descended to its normal position.

Normal swallowing is highly regulated by the afferent and efferent functions of the cranial nerves (Figure 2) in coordination with a postulated swallowing reflex center. This reflex center is located in the medulla where the pharyngeal constrictor muscles are controlled,[7] and possibly in the pons.[8] The highly complex action of the swallowing reflex described above is normally a precise and stable response pattern. As stated before, although it is centrally regulated, swallowing also requires some peripheral initiation (such as palatal stimulation by light touch or water) to proceed. Finally, bilateral innervation of the swallowing mechanisms allows contralateral swallowing to proceed normally in the case of unilateral brainstem lesions.[4]

SWALLOWING DISORDERS

In the adult, there are two major categories of swallowing disorders: neurologic, involving the nervous system, and mechanical involving the oral, pharyngeal, or laryngeal structures. The neurologic disorders may be divided into myogenic, affecting smooth or striated muscles; neurogenic, affecting the central nervous system centers, spinal cord, and peripheral nerves; and psychogenic involving primary or associated psychological or emotional causes. Mechanical disorders result most often from carcinoma or surgical resections secondary to carcinoma. Additional causes include acute inflammation, trauma, and macroglossia (abnormally large tongue). A more detailed overview of the following disorders may be found in Groher.[4]

Neurogenic Disorders

Neurologic disorders of the cortex secondary to CVA or vascular disorders may affect voluntary motor and reflex pathways. Dysphagia, drooling, choking, impaired gag, and release of primitive reflexes (rooting, suck, snout) may result. In brainstem strokes, the swallowing center itself may be affected, usually resulting in failure of the cricopharyngeal muscle to relax. Cricopharyngeal achalasia, as this failure of the relaxation phase is called, may be due to incomplete or uncoordinated movements of the pharyngeal muscle sequence. The resulting complaints are food sticking in the back of the throat, the need to swallow or clear the throat repeatedly, hoarseness, or coughing.[5,9]

Cranial nerves V, VII, IX, X, and XII also originate in the pons. Cranial nerve involvement may result in sensory and motor impairment of the face, lips, tongue, and oral cavity. Symptoms may include difficulty or delayed swallow, drooling, food retention in the side of the mouth (squirreling), facial droop, tongue weakness, and impairment of the gag and palatal reflexes.[10]

Parkinson's Disease is a movement disorder which commonly results in delayed swallow, irregular epiglottal movements, and impaired motility of the esophagus. In amyotrophic lateral sclerosis, mononeuron degeneration of the brainstem may cause secondary speech and swallowing impairments, while cranial nerve involvement may lead to weakness of the tongue and palate and laryngeal disorders.

The cranial nerves may be affected by acquired disorders such as infection, carcinoma, leukemia, and lymphoma. Although the most critical cranial neuropathy is involvement of the tenth cranial nerve, lesions of the V, VII, IX, and XII nerves may all contribute to dysphagia symptoms.

Neurodevelopmental disorders, most commonly cerebral palsy, may affect swallowing. While not progressive, the swallowing problems are generally related to neuromuscular incoordination, abnormal muscle tone, and weakness or paralysis of swallowing-related structures.

Myogenic Disorders

Myogenic disorders, myopathies and myotonias (including dystrophies) may involve the tongue and pharyngeal muscles and esophageal peristalsis, with aspiration a common problem. Myasthenia gravis may present with laryngeal weakness and dysphagia, and dysarthria caused by impaired conduction of the myoneural junction of striated muscle. Esophageal motility disorders may result from any of the neurologic disorders described. Usually the esophageal sphincter muscles are involved, often accompanied by sticking sensations and the need to wash solid foods down with fluids. Raymond's disease and scleroderma may affect the esophagus with smooth as well as striated muscle involvement.

Psychogenic Disorders

Psychogenic causes of dysphagia may be primary as in globus hystericus (a lump in the throat), secondary as in peptic ulcer disease, or associated to specific abnormalities in Plummer-Vinson syndrome. Some of these do not actually interfere with the act of swallowing or may involve other areas of the gastrointestinal tract. As organic causes may be involved, a physical examination is indicated.[4]

Mechanical Disorders

Groher[4] summarizes some of the symptoms shared by neurologic and mechanical dysphagia: drooling, mastication difficulty, oral and pharynageal pooling, prolonged duration of swallowing, difficulty directing food into the esophagus, and aspiration. The difference between the two types is in cause and structure. In mechanical disorders, the oral and pharyngeal structures are directly altered, most often due to surgery resulting from cancer. In addition, acute inflammation (bacterial, chemical, viral, or traumatic) may cause pain and discomfort on swallowing. These are usually treated and controlled in a short time if identified early. Macroglossia can interfere with the tongue's ability to maneuver the bolus; this condition may be secondary to lymphatic obstruction after surgery or irradiation, hyperthyroidism, and mongolism among others.

Carcinoma of the oral, pharyngeal, laryngeal, and esophageal structures and resulting irradiation and/or surgery comprise the most prevalent cause of mechanical dysphagia. The extent of the dysphagia is dependent partially on the extent of surgical excision. Oral lesions and resulting resections may involve the tongue, floor of the mouth, tonsils, soft palate, mandible, and/or maxilla. The impairments most common to this group are related to mastication, formulating and transporting the bolus posteriorly, and the timing of swallowing in relation to prolonged mastication. Partial and total laryngectomies frequently result in swallowing dysfunction and aspiration. The extent of the problem is partly dependent on whether the base of the tongue is preserved, if there is sufficient glottic closure, the presence of cricopharyngeal dysfunction, and the additional need for irradiation. Pre- or postoperative irradiation may produce complicating side effects such as oral and pharyngeal inflammation and pain, drying out of the mucosa, reduced and thickened saliva, taste changes, and loss of appetite.

Finally, mechanical obstructions may result during cervical spine disease from pressure on the esophagus, and during tracheostomy tube use from interference with the rise of the larynx. Cuff-type tracheostomy tubes may carry the additional risk of overinflation which causes pressure on the tracheosophageal wall.

EVALUATION

Although the evaluation of the dysphagic individual should be a team effort involving the medical services of neurology, otolaryngology, and gastroenterology in diagnosis and medical management, nursing, dietary, speech pathology, physical therapy, and pulmonary services, as indicated, the occupational therapist can play a prominent role in the functional pre-feeding assessment. A dysphagia evaluation is indicated for any individual suspected or known to have a swallowing impairment or related disorder (such as orofacial weakness and sensory loss), particularly in the presence of one of the diagnoses discussed above.

Any of the following symptoms may indicate the need for closer examination: coughing or choking on food or saliva, difficulty maneuvering of food in the mouth, excessive drooling, food retention in the mouth or pharyngeal recesses (determined by radiography), prolonged or obvious effort during swallowing, complaints of pain, discomfort or obstruction during swallowing, or presence of a feeding tube. If any of these symptoms is coupled with an absent or hyperactive gag reflex, dysarthric speech, or unusual respiration, evaluation is also indicated.

The primary contraindication for feeding, aside from medical or surgical problems, is poor mental status. Most often a concern with the neurologic population, the presence of lethargy, confusion, and poor cognitive abilities (distractibility, impaired judgment, perseveration) may pose a risk for safe oral feeding. The goal of evaluation and treatment is to achieve as normal a feeding regimen as possible without the risk of aspiration.

As this author has published a dysphagia evaluation format in a previous article,[11] a detailed description will not be repeated. For the benefit of the reader, however, a general review of the categories to be covered in a dysphagia evaluation is presented.

History-taking should include information about the onset of the swallowing difficulty, past eating habits and weight changes, medical and surgical history, medications, and use of dentures. Chart review will usually provide important information on current status, including respiratory status, communication status (speech or voice changes), current food or liquid intake, dietary restrictions, presenting complaints, and incidents of aspiration or attempts at feeding. On physical examination, the evaluator tests for normal reflexes (gag, cough, swallow) and abnormal or primitive reflexes (rooting, suck, snout, bite, and postural reflexes) particularly in neurologic impairment; appearance of teeth, gums, and tongue; strength and symmetry of the neck muscles, facial muscles, jaw, lips, and tongue; sensation on the face, lips, tongue, and palate (including taste); and voluntary movements and praxis of oral and facial structures including presence of spontaneous and voluntary swallows. It should be noted that abnormalities may increase with age in lip posture, masticatory muscles, tongue function, and on a rare occasion swallowing.[12]

Radiographic studies including cine- and video-fluoroscopy may be needed in cases of progressive or chronic dysphagia or when mechanical causes are suspected. Bolus transport in the pharyngeal and upper esophageal phases can be observed, indicating pharyngeal muscle involvement or obstruction of the cricopharyngeal muscle.[5,9] Motion fluoroscopy may also be of critical importance in detecting aspiration which may otherwise be unobserved. In a study of fifteen patients with neurologic dysphagia affecting pharyngeal function, the most common symptoms of aspiration (coughing, impaired gag reflex, and hoarse voice quality) were not completely reliable. Interestingly, subjects who could cough to command still did not always cough upon aspiration. Thus, despite the expense and risk of fluoroscopy it may be indicated in the presence of other suggestive clinical observations listed above.[13]

TREATMENT

As with many treatment methods, a well-executed evaluation may also be the first treatment session. The strength test provides an initial exercise period, and the trial swallows allow the therapist to continue with a food trial or other techniques to facilitate a swallow reflex. Whereas the functional pre-feeding assessment may be applied to both neurologic and mechanical feeding disorders, treatment procedures differ. The treatment discussion will first address general management principles. This will be followed by specific treatment suggestions for the two types of disorders.

General Management

The treatment environment should be quiet, well-lit, and distraction-free. For the dysphagic who is less alert, stimulation should be provided which is planned and well-ordered, such as by lighting, color, and therapist's voice and manner.[14] Feeding sessions should be scheduled at a favorable time of day when the client is hungry and well-rested. As much as possible, individual food preferences, eating routines, and personal habits should be considered. The client must be made comfortable and proper positioning utilized. This consists of an upright and symmetrical posture with the head slightly forward (chin tucked) and in midline position to provide best alignment of the alimentary tract during and after eating (15–30 minutes). Teeth and gums should be cleaned well and dried secretions removed with lemon-glycerine swabs or a washcloth. Denture-wearers are advised to continue wearing their dentures unless increased sensory stimulation necessitates temporary removal. The first feeding is best planned for nasogastric (N-G) tube users when the tube has been removed. If tube feedings are required, the N-G tube may be used intermittently or a small diameter pliable tube utilized. The latter is chosen to minimize the discomfort and possible inhibition of the gag reflex which may occur with a larger-diameter tube.

Treatment for Neurologic Disorders

Due to the particular problems of the neurologically-impaired population, special considerations and preparations must be addressed before and during the first feeding session. In upper motor neuron lesions, abnormal postural reflexes may be exhibited. Proper positioning can help to inhibit postural as well as abnormal oral reflexes.[15] Increasing flexion at the hip and knee joints and keeping any placement of pillows low on the shoulders or back (rather than behind the head) will avoid eliciting the tonic labyrinthine reflex and resulting neck extension. If optimal positioning is difficult to achieve due to problems of abnormal tone, inhibition and facilitation techniques should precede feeding.

If sensory impairment is present, increasing the individual's awareness through cognitive cues, the use of mirrors, and frequent checks for residual food is a necessary safety measure. To compensate for oral sensory loss, food may be initially directed to the more sensitive areas of the mouth. Farber recommends several methods to reduce *hypersensitivity*,[15] such as maintained pressure to the perioral area (placing the therapist's finger horizontally across the maxilla between the nose and upper lip), pressure to cheeks and temples if needed, and then maintained pressure to the dorsum of the tongue with a rubber seizure stick in the midline one-third of the way back on the tongue. Lip-shaped thermoplastic material may be molded to a padded tongue blade for this purpose.

Since this author has previously reported[11] on numerous techniques to strengthen oral and facial musculature, facilitate normal reflexes and inhibit abnormal reflexes, these methods will not be repeated. An interesting study was Huffman's use of biofeedback on the orbicularis oris muscle,[16] in which retraining lip movements resulted in greater and faster gains during mirror exercises when they were combined with EMG feedback. It should be noted that strengthening exercises may be contraindicated in some degenerative neurological diseases.[4]

Although water is highly stimulating to the swallow reflex, it is poorly controlled by neurologic dysphagics and frequently results in choking. In radiographic studies, aspiration is found to occur most readily when liquids are swallowed and least readily when semisolids are swallowed by neurologic dysphagics.[12] Food selection for test swallows should consider taste, temperature, bulk or texture, and odor. Initial food items should be appealing and safe in order to trigger the weak swallowing reflex. Small amounts of crushed ice or ice popsicles utilize water in a more controllable form for early swallow tests. Banana- or vanilla-flavored popsicles stimulate sucking[15] while the cold temperature is stimulating to oral sensory receptors. If the ice leads to choking, a water-moistened lollip may be tried. Sucking on a sweet-flavored lollip will stimulate salivation and taste receptors for swallowing. If aspiration is suspected, sugar-based items should be avoided as they increase the risk of aspiration pneumonia. If choking recurs, other foods should not be attempted.

When test swallows result in consistent and effective swallows (examiner should watch or feel the throat for the complete rise of the larynx on swallowing), trial foods may be initiated. Miller and Groher[4] suggest gelatins, especially when made with less water or blenderized to a whipped state, in medium-sized spoonsful (about 15 cc).[4] The spoon is placed firmly down on the center of the tongue to encourage active lip closure and removal of the food.[17] The spoon is always introduced in midline position at a low height to maintain correct head positioning. The mouth is checked for residual food. If the patient cannot clear the mouth by swallowing or spitting it out, the mouth should be cleared with a swab. During initial feeding sessions only one or two spoonsful may be tolerated before fatigue or deterioration is noted. Small portions offered more frequently may be desirable.

The food progression can proceed from jelled or blenderized foods (not bland, tepid purees, please) to soft solids (poached or scrambled eggs), thick liquids (thickened soups, nectars), early chewing foods (soft cooked vegetables, macaroni), and finally liquids and solids. Food choices should be individualized to the subject's tolerance and observed capabilities. Items to avoid are sticky foods (white bread), dry foods (mashed potatoes), mucous producers (chocolate, milk products), and foods that fall apart (crackers, applesauce).[4] Drinking can be initiated in full shallow cups to discourage tilting the head back. Liquid should be sipped, not poured into the mouth, without removing the cup between every sip.[7]

Cognitive cues may be needed by neurologic patients who can direct their efforts cortically despite a loss of automatic control over swallowing. By exercising voluntary control over their musculature, they may re-learn or consciously direct the swallowing process.

Cues to hold the breath while swallowing, swallow, and exhale or clear the throat by coughing can be useful. Intact cognitive skills may facilitate rehabilitation.[4]

Several studies have been published which describe successful courses of treatment with neurologic dysphagia. Harris and Murry[18] present a case study of a dysarthric and aphagic individual who was able to improve in articulation and resume an oral diet following a modified speech therapy program. The treatment program focused on abdominal breathing, velopharyngeal and glottac closure, tongue and lip range of motion and strength, which are all needed in normal swallowing. An intensive exercise program included coughing, producing hard sounds ("K") for glottic closure, resisted sucking and blowing through a straw, and isometric and isotonic tongue exercises. Griffin[19] who also utilizes speech exercises, and Heimlich[20] describe swallowing training techniques which include cognitive instruction coupled with manipulation of diet. In both methods, the authors break down the swallowing sequence into steps for practice and mastery. Griffin relies specifically on verbal commands to retrain the swallowing sequence (raise tongue tip to roof of mouth—think about swallowing—swallow).

In summary, Winstein[21] reports the results of a retrospective chart review of head-injured patients admitted to a rehabilitation facility. Of the 25% who exhibited swallowing or oral-motor impairments on admission, 94% of these individuals eventually became successful oral feeders. The programs utilized included sensory stimulation or desensitization of oral and facial structures, muscle facilitation techniques, and diet manipulation. Of those who remained non-oral feeders, the most frequent problems interfering with therapy were poor cognition and oral motor control.

Treatment for Mechanical Disorders

There are two major differences in treatment between neurologic and mechanical dysphagia. Whereas the neurologic group often chokes on clear liquids, the mechanical dysphagics may swallow liquids without difficulty. Rather, this group usually will complain that solid foods "get stuck" in the throat. Secondly, whereas the emphasis for the former group is on therapeutic exercises, muscle reeducation, and reflex stimulation, the emphasis for the latter is on medical or surgical intervention followed by compensation with adaptive utensils and eating techniques. This usually involves for the therapist choosing a mechanical device to aid in transporting the bolus through the oral cavity.

Two of these devices reported in Groher[4] are the glossectomy feeding spoon (available from Fred Sammons, Inc., Brookfield, Ill.) and the 50- or 60-cc. syringe. (See Figures 3 and 4.) The glossectomy feeding spoon transports the bolus to the oropharynx when the tongue cannot due to resection. It is recommended when there is little risk of aspiration and when at least 50% of the tongue is removed so it does not interfere with the device. Blenderized or finely chopped foods, easiest to handle[22] and not requiring mastication, are placed as far back in the oral cavity as possible toward the area of best sensation or tongue mass. The sliding mechanism is then used to push the food off the spoon for deposit onto the base of the tongue.

The 50- or 60-cc. catheter-tipped syringe with 15-cm. extension of connecting tubing is recommended for tongue paresis or less than 50% tongue resection. In using this device, the distal tip of the extension tubing is placed in the area of the mouth for easiest handling, such as on the unresected portion of the tongue. Liquids and thin purees may be administered with the device.

Dry mouth caused by irradiation or medication should be alleviated prior to eating with lemon-glycerine swabs, or synthetic saliva. The upright position is maintained except when, if the risk of aspiration is slight, bolus transport problems are compounded by heaving drooling. Then a semi-reclining position (about 50°) may be maintained as long as the head and trunk are in the same plane.[4] As with neurologic dysphagics, cognitive cues may be utilized to avoid aspiration and clear the airway (e.g., inhale-swallow-exhale/cough/reswallow). Generally, patients with cognitive skills intact are better candidates for rehabilitation.

Heimlich and O'Connor[23] describe several patients whose physical defects prevented swallowing of food and led to long-term tube feedings. After surgery to correct the defects, they remained unable to swallow. The authors suggest the patients had forgotten how to swallow. Following a methodology similar to that which Heimlich developed for CVA patients as described above, he found they were able to relearn the swallowing process.

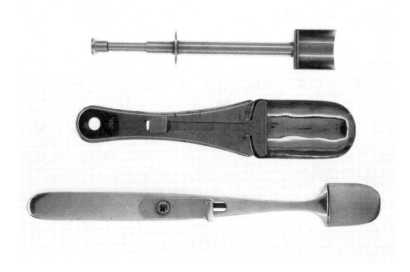

FIGURE 3. (Top) Commercially available glossectomy feeding spoon. (Middle) Cooking measuring spoon that should *not* be used for feeding. (Bottom) Glossectomy feeding spoon available for eligible military veterans. (Reprinted from Groher with permission of author and publisher.)

CONCLUSIONS AND SUMMARY

Active rehabilitation of the adult with dysphagia has been long in its actualization. While many of the methods such as reflex facilitation or inhibition have been borrowed from pediatric use, others such as cognitive cues are being developed with the adult in mind. The benefits of dysphagia treatment programs extend far beyond the medical benefits or reducing the risk of aspiration while adequately maintaining oral nutrition. Resuming normal eating behavior offers personal satisfaction to the patient who is in control of this pleasurable and basic function. Furthermore, it has been noted that other social habits are resumed following a successful program.[18]

In reviewing normal and pathological swallowing behavior, the therapist is cautioned to obtain medical clearance for all evaluations and treatments introduced. Since the physician is ultimately responsible for the patient's safety in the event of potentially life-

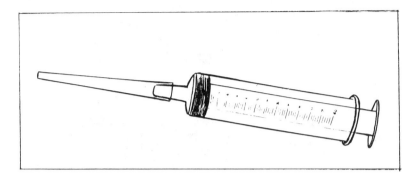

FIGURE 4. Catheter-tipped 60-cc. Syringe with extension device of pliable tubing.

threatening aspiration, as well as for all dietary orders, it is well to coordinate the dysphagia program with the medical team.

The intent of this paper was to present to the practitioner some of the important treatment techniques and considerations aimed at the adult dysphagic population. When coupled with earlier writings on evaluation and treatment, this should provide the clinician with a good foundation in this area of practice. It was also the author's intent, however, to discriminate between the neurological and mechanical causes of dysphagia and among the many diagnoses in each category. It should be understood that dysphagia is not one entity, but can present with a variety of symptomatologies that should be treated with individualized approaches. Finally, it is hoped that by continuing to gather evaluation and treatment methods for the dysphagic population, the reader will be motivated to test the effectiveness of these measures in clinical research.

BIBLIOGRAPHY

1. Donner MW: Swallowing mechanism and neuromuscular disorders. *Sem Reontgenol* IX (4): 273–282, 1974

2. Larsen GL: Conservative management for incomplete dysphagia paralytica. *Arch Phys Med Rehabil* 54: 180–185, April 1973

3. Roueche JR: Dysphagia: An Assessment and Management Program for the Adult. Minneapolis: Sister Kenny Institute, 1980

4. Groher ME, ed: Dysphagia: Diagnosis and Management. Stoneham, Ma: Butterworth Publishers, 1984

5. Schultz A, Niemtzow P, Jacobs S, Naso F: Dysphagia associated with cricopharyngeal dysfunction. *Arch Phys Med Rehabil* 60: 381–6, 1979

6. Mansson I, Sandberg N: Oro-pharyngeal sensitivity and elicitation of swallowing in man. *Octa Otolaryngol* 79: 140–145, 1975

7. Doty RW, Richmond WH, Storey AT: Effect of medullary lesions on coordination of deglutition. *Exp Neurol* 17: 91–106, 1967

8. Holstege G, Graveland G, Bijker-Biemond C, Schuddeboom I: Location of Motoneurous Innervating Soft Palate, Pharynx, and Upper Esophagus. Anatomical evidence for a possible swallowing center in the pontine reticular formation. *Brain Behav Evol* 23 (1–2): 47–62, 1983

9. Dietz F, Logemann JA, Sahgal V, Schnid FR: Cricopharyngeal muscle dysfunction in the differential diagnosis of dysphagia in polymyositis. *Arth Rheum* 23: 491–495, 1980

10. Mysack ED: Dysarthria and oropharyngeal reflexology: A review. *J Speech Hear Disord* 28(3): 252–260, 1963

11. Silverman EH, Elfant IL: Dysphagia: An evaluation and treatment program for the adult. *Am J Occup Ther* 33: 382–392, 1979

12. Age, Masticatory ability and swallowing, *Nutr Rev* 41 (11) 344–346, 1983

13. Linden P, Siebens AA: Dysphagia: Predicting laryngeal penetration. *Arch Phys Med Rehabil* 64: 281–284, 1983

14. Trombly CA, Scott AD: Occupational Therapy for Physical Dysfunction. Baltimore: Williams & Wilkins, 1979

15. Farber SD: Neurorehabilitation: A Multi-Sensory Approach. Philadelphia: WB Saunders, 1982

16. Huffman AL: Biofeedback treatment of orofacial dysfunction: A preliminary study. *Am J Occup Ther* 32: 149–152, 1978

17. Mueller HA: Facilitating Feeding and Pre-Speech. In Physical Therapy Services in the Developmental Disabilities, PH Pearson, CA Williams, editors, Springfield, IL: Charles C. Thomas: 283–310, 1972

18. Harris B, Murry T: Dysarthria and aphagia: A case study of neuromuscular treatment. *Arch Phys Med Rehabil* 65(7): 408–412, 1984

19. Griffin KM: Swallowing training for dysphagic patients. *Arch Phys Med Rehabil* 55: 467–470, 1974

20. Heimlich HJ: Rehabilitation of swallowing after stroke. *Ann Otol Rhinol Laryngol* 92 (4:1): 357–359, 1983

21. Winstein CJ: Neurogenic dysphagia: Frequency, progression, and outcome in adults following head injury. *Phys Ther* 63(12): 1992–1997, 1983

22. Miller RM, Groher ME: Evaluation and Management of Neuromuscular and Mechanical Swallowing Disorders In Eggart G. Milianti Fed: Dysarthria, Dysphonia, Dysphagia. Chicago, Biolinguistics Clinical Institutes, 1982

23. Heimlich HJ, O'Connor TW: Relearning the swallowing process. *Ann Otol Rhinol Laryngol* 88(6): 794–797, 1979

An Occupational Therapy Program for Patients With Swallowing Dysfunction Following Cancer Treatment

Laura Cleary, OTR

ABSTRACT. Eating, the intimate activity of daily living, carries with it many emotional, social and physical implications. Medical treatment of patients with cancers of the head and neck is frequently radical and almost certainly impacts on the patient's ability to eat. This paper outlines an occupational therapy program for patients with swallowing dysfunction following treatment for cancers of the head and neck. Discussed in this paper are the medical treatments particular to cancer treatment that directly affect swallowing function, along with evaluation and treatment by the occupational therapist. The paper concludes with a case study.

The City of Hope is a medical and research center specializing in the care of persons suffering catastrophic and debilitating disease, the majority of whom are diagnosed with cancer. As part of the interdisciplinary team, the Department of Occupational Therapy plays an active role in the care and treatment of these patients. The purpose of this paper is to describe the occupational therapy program at the City of Hope for the treatment of patients with swallowing dysfunction following treatment for cancers of the head and neck. Medical treatments of head and neck cancers are frequently radical and may include surgical excision and chemo-

Laura Cleary is a staff occupational therapist, Rehabilitation Department, City of Hope National Medical Center, Duarte, CA, 1981-present. She graduated in 1979 with a BS degree in Occupational Therapy from York College of CUNY, Jamaica, NY.

The author wishes to acknowledge the assistance of Mrs. June Benes and Ms. Susan Treat in typing the manuscript.

This article appears jointly in *Occupational Therapy for People With Eating Dysfunctions* (The Haworth Press, Inc., 1986) and *Occupational Therapy in Health Care*, Volume 3, Number 2 (Summer 1986).

23

therapy, radiation therapy, or any combination of them. These treatments will almost certainly have some impact on the patient's ability to eat. The intimate activity of daily living, eating, carries with it many emotional, social, and physical implications. Dysfunction in this area must be addressed to assure that the person so affected has maximum potential for quality of life.

At the City of Hope, prior to the patient undergoing a surgical procedure for head and neck cancer, a conference is held with the members of the interdisciplinary team, the patient and his family. The team will generally consist of a nurse coordinator, discharge planner, occupational therapist, physical therapist, social worker, speech therapist and dietician. The physician has met with the patient prior to this meeting to explain the proposed treatment. At the conference, the surgical procedure is again reviewed in layman's terms allowing time for questions. Persons/staff from each discipline then have an opportunity to explain their role in the patient's post-operative treatment. At this time, the occupational therapist can discuss the anticipated swallowing/feeding problems, treatment planned and expected outcomes. Generally, these pre-surgical meetings help to alleviate many fears and concerns of both the patient and family. Having this information prior to surgery seems to have a very positive influence on the patient's ability to participate fully in his post-operative rehabilitative course. It also gives the occupational therapist an opportunity to assess the patient's functional status, coping style, and support systems prior to the surgery when he can more fully participate in discussions.

Patients who undergo radiation therapy as their primary treatment are usually referred for occupational therapy services after swallowing problems have been identified.

TREATMENTS THAT IMPACT ON SWALLOWING FUNCTION

The treatments for cancers of the head and neck are frequently damaging to the anatomical structures involved in the performance of chewing and swallowing. In order to assess the needs of these patients, the therapist must be familiar with the normal mechanism of swallowing as well as with specific treatments that impact directly on these structures. The following are descriptions of some of the procedures and treatments commonly performed in the treatment of patients with head and neck cancers that impact directly on swallowing function.

Surgical Excision

When surgery is performed for the removal of a cancerous tumor, the surgeon must not only excise the tumor but also a "clear margin" of tissue free of cancerous cells around it. Due to their close proximity, excision rarely involves just one structure. When evaluating swallowing function, the cumulative effects of multi-structure involvement must be considered. A general rule of thumb to follow in assessing the surgical patient is the following: when 50% or less of a structure is resected, mild to moderate impairment of that structure's function can be expected. Fifty percent or more resection will result in significant impairment to total dysfunction.[6]

A *radical neck dissection* (RND) involves the removal of the cervical lymph node chain, resection of the spinal accessory nerve, sternocleidomastoid, omohyoid, posterior digastric, and styloid muscles, as well as branches of the internal jugular vein.[9] Other than the discomfort from the surgical incision and post-operative swelling, a RND does not generally cause long term swallowing dysfunction.

A *laryngectomy* may be total or subtotal depending upon the extent of tumor involvement. A total laryngectomy involves removal of the entire laryngeal complex and the creation of a permanent tracheostomy.[9] Because the trachea is diverted to an opening at the neck and no further communication exists with the oral pharynx, no aspiration of food into lung is possible unless a fistula exists between the wall of the trachea and pharynx. However, the possibility of scarring in the pharynx causing pocketing or stricture may impair the patient's ability to swallow all textures and normal volumes of food. This condition may require mechanical dilatation of the pharynx by the physician.

A *supraglottic laryngectomy* involves the removal of the hyoid bone, epiglottis, aryepiglottic folds, and the false vocal cords.[9] This procedure leaves only the true vocal cords as a protective mechanism against aspiration. Patients having this procedure are at high risk of aspiration and must be instructed in techniques to protect their airway. This will be discussed later.

The creation of a *tracheostomy* may be permanent (as in total laryngectomy) or temporary. It is common in surgeries of the head and neck, secondary to the amount of swelling involved and the resulting constriction of the airway. A puncture is created through the neck just above the sternal notch to the trachea. A tracheostomy tube is frequently inserted into the tracheostoma to maintain the airway patency and provide access for tracheal suctioning. Tracheostomy tubes placed in surgery patients are usually cuffed. The cuff is an inflatable plastic ring at the distal end of the tracheostomy tube. When the ring or cuff is inflated, it applies gentle pressure against the tracheal wall thus preventing secretions or food from being aspirated into the lungs. The presence of a tracheostomy tube usually is not directly a cause for aspiration. Because of the position of the tube, however, it may cause a very uncomfortable sensation of pulling when the larynx must elevate during swallowing or the cuff may put excessive pressure on the wall of the pharynx.

A *pharyngectomy* may include any portion of the oro, naso, or hypopharynx.[9] Again, the extent of the resection and the effects on adjacent structures will determine the functional loss. Scarring and resulting stricture in the pharynx may contribute to swallowing dysfunction.

A *glossectomy* involves resection of any portion of the tongue. The degree of functional loss will depend greatly on the location of resection (anterior, posterior, or base of tongue) and the technique the surgeon uses to reconstruct the excised area. This procedure obviously will have some effect on tongue mobility and strength. A decrease in mobility often results in poor bolus propulsion and may contribute to aspiration due to poor bolus control resulting in premature spillage of materials into the pharynx before the swallowing reflex is triggered and adequate tracheal closure is attained. Decreased ability to elevate the posterior tongue may also play a part in decreased triggering of the swallowing reflex.[6] Resection of the base of the tongue may cause scarring that can greatly impair the ability of the epiglottis to adequately close off the airway during swallowing.

Palatectomy may include any portion of the hard or soft palate. When a portion of the palate is excised, use of an oral prosthesis is necessary to compensate for loss of the mechanical barrier up against which the bolus of food is propelled by the tongue. Loss of the soft palate is not as easily compensated for by prosthesis as compared to the hard palate. Loss of the soft palate may result in difficulty in propulsion of bolus from the oral cavity and also cause a tendency for nasal reflux of food. Extension of pharyngeal or soft palate resection to the faucial arch may impair the triggering of the reflexive swallow and subsequently contribute to aspiration. The anterior faucial pillars are considered the most sensitive structures for elicitation of the swallowing reflex. If the faucial pillars are included in the resection, stimulation of the swallowing reflex is decreased or absent. The swallowing reflex triggers the larynx to close and protect the airway. If the swallowing reflex is not triggered the individual will most likely attempt to compensate with excessive tongue movement to propel the bolus into the pharynx. In these cases the possibility of materials entering the open airway is increased.

Due to large sections of tissue that are frequently excised in head and neck surgeries, *myocutaneous flaps* are utilized for reconstruction of the site of resection. A myocutaneous flap includes muscle tissue and an island of overlying skin with the attachment as well as blood supply left intact. The flap is then moved to the area to be reconstructed.[2] Myocutaneous grafts are frequently used to reconstruct the floor of the mouth or pharynx. Although a graft can replace the bulk of the tissue resected, it cannot replace the function of the structure.

Feeding tubes are frequently placed when long term swallowing difficulties are anticipated. They do not significantly impair swallowing function. The presence of a nasogastric tube is cumbersome and is sometimes irritating to the nasopharyngeal tract. In rare cases where there is pharyngeal stricture or decreased pharyngeal peristalsis, the presence of a tube may produce a mechanical obstruction.

Radiation Therapy

Radiation therapy is used as a primary treatment for head and neck cancers as well as an adjuvant to surgical excision. The effects of radiation treatment may take several weeks to surface. The symptoms may last 4–6 weeks. Some tissue damage may be permanent. Tissue erythema, swelling, and fibrosis are common. Radiated tissue has poor healing capability due to damage of the capillary beds and is prone to development of salivary fistula in the oral cavity. Xerostomia or dry mouth is common, as are dental problems. The constant production of thick 'ropey' secretions that require frequent suctioning is a definite management problem in swallowing training. Increased fatigue is also a factor to be considered.[8]

Chemotherapy

Chemotherapy is generally used as an adjuvant to radiation therapy or surgical excision, usually for control of metastatic disease. Common side effects that impact on swallowing function include; generalized weakness and fatigue, anorexia, nausea, and a sore, ulcerated mouth or throat. Taste blindness and food aversions are also sometimes experienced.[8]

EVALUATION

Referral of a patient to occupational therapy for swallowing function assessment and training may occur at various stages of medical treatment. The post-surgical patient is referred by the physician when adequate healing and reduction of edema have taken place. In general, this is 1–2 weeks after surgery. Patients receiving radiation or chemotherapy are also referred after acute symptoms such as erythema or mucositis have subsided.

Prior to initiation of the functional assessment, a thorough medical chart review is completed to determine the present status of the patient and factors that will impact on swallowing function. Special note is paid to prior treatments, a history of dysphagia, weight loss, or general weakness and fatigue. Present diet management is also identified. If tube feedings are being done, arrangements are made for therapy sessions to be scheduled prior to feedings. The respiratory status and management (i.e., tracheostomy) are identified. If the patient has required frequent suctioning or does not have a productive cough, and a high aspiration risk is anticipated, arrangements are made for a nurse to be present at the initial session for tracheal suctioning as needed.

BEDSIDE ASSESSMENT

At the bedside, assessment of range of motion, strength, coordination and sensitivity of the oral structures is completed. This includes evaluation of labial function, lingual function, soft palate function, oral reflexes and laryngeal function. The patient's ability to produce a strong cough is assessed as well as his level of alertness and ability to follow instruction. The confines of this paper will not allow for detailed descriptions of the functional assessment of the structures involved in the swallowing mechanism. However, this can be obtained from the references listed.[1,6] A history of the patient's eating patterns and any specific swallowing problems from the patient is taken. Exploration of the patient's feelings about eating, his lifestyle and goals are imperative for successful treatment planning.

When evaluating a patient who has already demonstrated symptoms of aspiration or when it is highly anticipated that due to structure involvement that he is at risk for aspiration, a videofluoroscopic study of swallowing function is completed (physicians order required). A videofluoroscopy is a radiographic study in which the patient swallows a small amount of barium and the fluoroscopic image is recorded on video film. This study provides information on bolus transit time, motility problems, and the amount and etiology of aspiration. This information can only be definitively obtained from radiographic study. During the study the occupational therapist is present, as appropriate suggestions are made regarding use of adaptive techniques such as positioning, airway control, or use of adaptive feeding devices. These techniques will be discussed later. The results of the study are reported to the managing physician who then makes the decision whether to continue with oral feedings. At City of Hope, the parameters outlined by Logemann are generally followed for initiating oral feedings. If the patient is aspirating on more than 10 percent of a barium texture (liquid, paste, or paste on a cookie), that texture should be eliminated from the diet.[6] If the study demonstrates significant aspiration with each bolus, the patient is placed on NPO (nothing by mouth) and is considered to be an unreasonable high risk for aspiration in oral feedings until function improves. Assuming the assessment and training can proceed after completion of a prepartory bedside assessment, swallowing trials are initiated. The patient is given small amounts of various consistencies of foods including; a puree (i.e., applesauce), a semi-solid (i.e., custard), a clear liquid (i.e., apple juice, 7-Up). Frequently if there is a question of the presence of a fistula or aspiration (particularly if a tracheostomy tube is in place), some food coloring is added to provide a contrast. With patients who have a tracheostomy, to assure a clear airway and oral cavity, oral and tracheal suctioning should be done. If the tracheostomy tube is cuffed it should be deflated during the assessment unless the physician orders otherwise. Tracheal suctioning following swallowing trials will also assist in detecting aspirations. This may require the assistance of the nursing staff for tracheal suctioning.

As the patient swallows, the therapist observes for the following: indication of aspiration, mechanical dysfunction, delayed or absent reflexive swallow, and presence of a fistula. At the bedside evaluation aspiration will usually result in coughing, choking, or throat clearing with the patient complaining of a "tickle" in the throat. The *phase* of swallowing in which the aspiration occurs is also noted. Aspiration *before* the swallow is initiated indicates that the airway was not yet closed when the bolus entered the hypopharynx. This is frequently due to poor tongue control of the bolus or a delayed or absent reflexive swallow. Aspiration *during* the swallow indicates laryngeal valving dysfunction such as poor adduction of the vocal cords. Aspiration *after* the swallow indicates that it has occurred after the larynx lowers and the airway opens. This may occur as a result of residual food pooling in the valleculae or pyriform sinus. Mechanical dysfunction may be seen as food pocketing at the side of the mouth secondary to poor tongue mobility or thicker foods' inability to pass through the pharynx due to scarring and stricture. Presence of the swallowing reflex may be detected by observing for elevation of the larynx or by gently palpating the laryngeal area.[6] Frequently the patient will struggle, attempting several times to swallow before the reflex triggers. Presence of a fistula is detected by leakage of food from a surgical incision. In the patients who have undergone a total laryngectomy leakage of food into the trachea also indicates a fistula.

TREATMENT PLANNING AND GOAL SETTING

Most patients who have undergone treatment for cancers of the head and neck will exhibit a combination of problems outlined in the previous section. Once the areas of dysfunction are identified, careful treatment planning is done. The results of the evaluation and the proposed treatment are discussed with the patient and, if possible, the family. At this time goals that are both realistic and appropriate are set. For some patients it is realistic to anticipate that they will return to a normal diet if their particular problems are generally responsive to therapeutic intervention (i.e., the patient who has undergone a supraglottic laryngectomy but is aspirating). Quite understandably the more extensive the procedures undergone the less likely it is that full function can be restored. A person who has undergone a partial pharyngectomy, hemi-mandibulectomy and floor of the mouth resection can not expect to eat steak again but may manage a diet of purees, some semi-solids, and liquids. It may also be appropriate to plan for a patient to remain on tube feeding while eating selected foods or drink for pleasure and satisfaction.

INTERVENTION

Occupational therapy intervention and treatment techniques for swallowing dysfunction vary with each individual case. They fall into the following general categories; techniques to protect the airway in swallowing, management of secretions, selection of appropriate food consistencies, positioning, facilitating reflexive swallow, exercises, use of adaptive equipment, family training, and most importantly emotional support and encouragement.

The ''supraglottic swallow'' is a technique taught to those who are aspirating due to poor airway closure. This technique teaches the patient to consciously hold his breath while swallowing and then coughing to clear the pharynx of any residual before breathing again.

Control of oral secretions in patients with head and neck cancers can be quite problematic. Prior to initiating any swallowing training the oral cavity and pharynx should be clear of excessive secretions. This may require vigorous coughing and suctioning. A portable suction unit for home use is recommended. Following radiation treatment saliva becomes thick and 'ropey,' making it difficult to expectorate it. To cut these secretions, the use of papaya juice, which contains the enzyme (papain) is helpful in breaking down saliva. Meat tenderizer contains this same enzyme and used in a gargle does a similar job.[5] As the swallowing mechanism normalizes, problems with secretions often lessen over time.

After completing the assessment, consistencies of foods that the patient can safely swallow are identified. The occupational therapist, dietician, and patient collaborate to formulate a diet. If special preparation is needed for foods, the patient or a family member are engaged in a training session in the occupational therapy kitchen. Sample menus and recipes are provided for home use.

Exercises to increase mobility, strength, and bolus control of the oral structures are often indicated. For patients who demonstrate poor airway closure during swallowing, exercises to increase adduction of tissue at the top of the airway are initiated.[6]

As simple a technique as positioning can result in significant improvement of swallowing function. By bringing the chin down, the vallecular space is widened which will allow the bolus to rest there long enough to facilitate triggering of the swallowing reflex. Positioning the head in this manner will allow the epiglottis to close the larynx more fully and offer better airway protection. If the patient is demonstrating decreased pharyngeal peristalsis it is helpful to turn toward the affected side to direct food to the stronger side. Alternating liquid and solid foods can also be useful. For poor oral control the head is tilted toward the stronger side.

Facilitory techniques such as quick icing to the neck muscles and direct stimulation to the anterior faucial arches to heighten or stimulate the reflexive swallow[6] are sometimes useful. However, these techniques seem to have only limited effect when treating the patient with cancer who has structural changes as opposed to one who is neurologically involved.

For the patient who demonstrates poor bolus control, adaptive equipment is used extensively. These pieces of equipment are used to place the bolus of food on the tongue in a position most easily swallowed. A 50 cc irrigating syringe (Figure 1) is available from most hospital unit supply carts. It can be used to feed both liquids and pureed foods. By attaching a length of rubber catheter on the tip this will enable the patient to place the bolus further back on the tongue. The semi-solid feeder (Figure 1) is a similar injection device. While the irrigating syringe can only be used several times before it must be discarded the semi-solid feeder is more durable and holds about a cup of pureed foods. The semi-solid feeder is available through Abbey Medical Supplies. The syringe bottle (Figure 1) is very helpful for drinking liquids. It is a soft plastic bottle that when squeezed will eject a stream of liquid from its spout that is angled at 90° allowing the patient to drink without throwing his head back. These bottles may be obtained from the hospital laboratory supplies department or at community sporting goods stores. The glossectomy spoon (Figure 2) is a long-handled spoon with a blade that can push the food off the spoon when the plunger

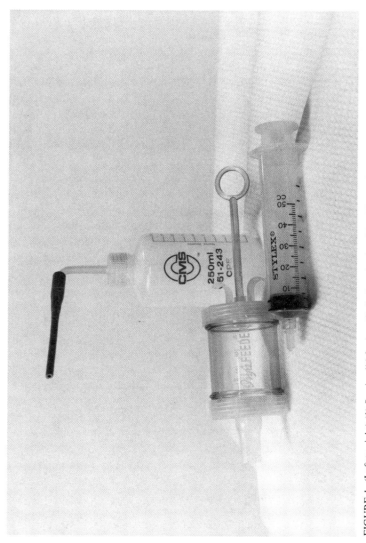

FIGURE 1. (Left to right) (1) Semi-solid feeder, (2) Syringe bottle with rubber catheter applied at tip, (3) 50 cc irrigating syringe.

is depressed. This device is used for thick pureed and semi-solid foods. The spoon pictured in Figure 2 is fabricated by the biomechanical instrumentations services at the City of Hope Medical Center. A similar spoon is commercially available through the Fred Sammons Co., Brookfield, Illinois.

Throughout the therapy period the patient's progress is monitored closely. The length of treatment may span from several days to several months. The patient is always given a home program to follow and his family is involved as much as possible in the program. When the patient is able to eat sufficient volumes of food to sustain his weight and nutritional needs and he is able to do so in a reasonable amount of time, the feeding tube can be removed and swallowing training discontinued. Of course not all patients are able to reach this point. When it is apparent that treatment is not effective or that the patient's progress has plateaued, treatment is discontinued. At this point the physician may consider placement of a more permanent feeding tube such as a gastrostomy tube. The following is a case study of a patient treated by Occupational Therapy for swallowing dysfunction at the City of Hope Medical Center.

Case Study—Mr. L

Mr. L is a 34 year old Hispanic male. In 1980 he underwent a wide local excision of a cancerous tumor of the right buccal mucosa. He then completed a course of radiation therapy to this area totaling 7100 rads. In 1984 there was a recurrence of the original tumor. He underwent a partial mandibulectomy, partial maxillectomy, partial resection of the soft palate and reconstruction with a trapezius myocutaneous flap. The facial nerve was also sacrificed in the resection. A nasogastric tube was placed for feeding. A permanent maxillary (hard palate) prosthesis was placed in surgery.

Prior to the second surgery a pre-surgical team conference was held with the patient and family. An individual occupational therapy evaluation was completed. Mr. L was found to have decreased mobility of the tempro-mandibular joint (3.5 cm mouth opening) and decreased bite pressure. He did not have difficulty eating a normal diet.

After his second surgery, the occupational therapy assessment identified the following problems; poor labial closure unilaterally, decreased oral sensation, decreased tongue mobility, poor palatal closure, decreased range of motion and pain of the tempro-

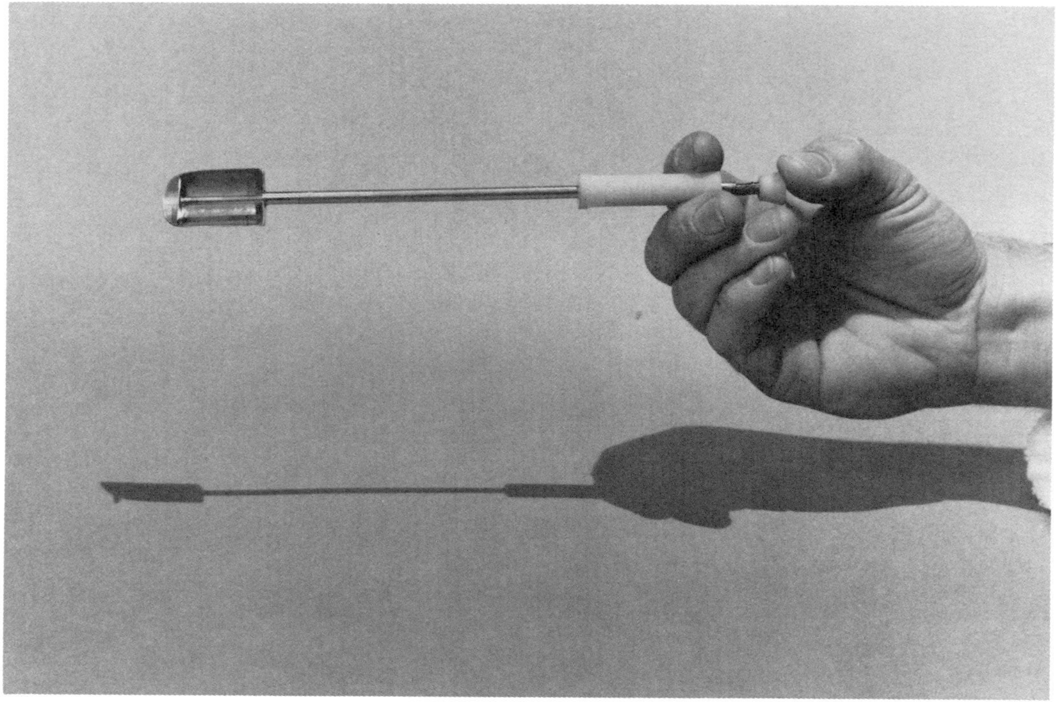

FIGURE 2. Glossectomy spoon.

mandibular joint. Combined, these deficits resulted in the following dysfunction; drooling and loss of food from the mouth, poor mastication and bolus propulsion, nasal reflux of food and occasional aspiration of food due to poor oral-motor control.

On the seventh post-operative day occupational therapy training was initiated. He was engaged in a graded program of exercises to increase mobility and strength of the tongue and jaw.

To decrease aspiration risk, Mr. L was instructed in a modified supraglottic swallowing technique. Foods were introduced gradually beginning with thick liquids (nectars, milkshakes) and semi-solid foods (custard, ice cream). This was later expanded to include all liquids, purees and easily masticated foods. To compensate for compromised oral-motor control a syringe bottle, semi-solid feeder, and glossectomy spoon were used. To assure that appropriate food textures and adequate caloric needs were met, the occupational therapist and dietician collaborated in assisting with menu selection. When arrangements were made for family members to bring in favorite ethnic dishes his intake improved significantly. Daily caloric counts were completed by the dietary department. Guidelines regarding appropriate food textures and preparation were discussed with the patient's wife.

After much effort the patient was able to maintain an adequate level of oral intake to sustain himself. The nasogastric tube was removed and shortly after he was discharged from the hospital. On a return out-patient visit one month following discharge, the patient reported that his eating was improving and he only occasionally needed the adaptive devices he was given. Although his menu was somewhat limited he was maintaining his weight and was pleased with the results.

SUMMARY

Occupational therapy for swallowing dysfunction in patients following treatment for head and neck cancers requires a thorough understanding of the swallowing function and of how medical procedures can impact on that function as well as careful assessment of individual needs and treatment. Due to the varying levels of involvement of these patients, treatment outcome is variable. To date no studies have been completed to measure the impact of occupational therapy programs on swallowing function following

cancer treatment; however this is planned for the future. Subjec-
tively, occupational therapy intervention has had positive impact on
improvement of quality of life.

REFERENCES

1. Abreu B: Physical Disabilities Manual, New York, Raven Press, 1981

2. Ariyan S: Further experiences with pectoralis major myocutaneous flap for the
immediate repair of defects from excisions of head and neck cancers, *Plast Reconstr Surg*,
November 1979

3. Dudgeon B, DeLisa J, Miller R: Head and neck cancer: A rehabilitation approach.
Am J Occ Ther, 34, 243–251, 1980

4. Larsen G L: Rehabilitation dysphagia mechanica, paralytica, pseudobulbar. *J Neuro
Nurs*, 8(1) 14–17, July 1976

5. Larsen G L: Rehabilitation for the patient with head and neck cancer, *Am J Nurs*, Jan
1982

6. Logeman J: *Evaluation and Treatment of Swallowing Disorders* San Diego College:
Hill Press, Inc., 1983

7. Netter F: *The Ciba Collection of Medical Illustrations, Volume 3: Digestive System*,
New York: Ciba Publishing Company, 1971

8. Rosenbaum E: *A Comprehensive Guide for Cancer Patients and Their Families*, Palo
Alto: Bull Publishing Company, 1980

9. Rubin P (Editor): *Clinical Oncology for Medical Students and Physicians: A
Multi-Disciplinary Approach, 5th Edition*: University of Rochester, American Cancer Society
Publications, 1978

10. Stuart M: Skin flaps and grafts after head and neck surgery. *Am J Nurs*, Aug 1978

11. Zimmerman O: Swallowing in acutely ill patients *Phys Ther*, 61/12, Dec 1981

The Role of Occupational Therapy in Planning Dining Programs in Institutions for the Frail Elderly

Suzanne Perket, OTR

ABSTRACT. Dining rooms in institutions for the frail elderly often reflect an atmosphere of speed, congestion, eating and being fed with minimal social interaction between residents and service personnel. The role of the occupational therapist in helping to create *a dining program* in such facilities is described. The importance of attention to individual resident needs, careful design of the setting and environment as well as planned strategies for conducting a dining program are emphasized. The key roles of staff and their attitudes are described.

In efforts to provide the aged with a proper diet, we fail to consider that it is not what the older person eats, but the interpersonal and environmental factors that will be the deciding factors in proper care.

Cornelia Beck, RN, PhD[1]

The American culture today places a strong emphasis on diet and nutrition. Most people like to eat with others, people they know and like. In other words, the meaning of mealtime goes beyond the simple intake of food. Mealtime is a social event that reflects one's values and habits. Dining is part of the social life of every

---

Suzanne Perket is President of St. Croix Therapy, a private practice occupational therapy service offering both consultation and direct service to acute and long term care institutions. She and her colleagues offer educational workshops in which practical solutions to common problems are offered to interdisciplinary staffs in many parts of the country. A particular program is entitled, *Back to the Table: A practical approach to long term care dining programs.* It is from that program and the author's philosophies that the present paper is developed.

This article appears jointly in *Occupational Therapy for People With Eating Dysfunctions* (The Haworth Press, Inc., 1986) and *Occupational Therapy in Health Care*, Volume 3, Number 2 (Summer 1986).

39

individual, the rich and poor of every nationality, every race, every age. For elderly persons who live in institutions, the interest in eating may be low or absent because of lack of stimulation in the dining environment, the absence of any of the 'cues' that are reminders of one's former habits and values. Yet, residents who have lost their interest in eating can often be remotivated to eat again and enjoy it if they are provided with the conditions in which eating is physically possible and there exists a social setting and environment that stimulates their desire to eat.

Health care providers too often fail to recognize that eating is more than simple self-maintenance, done three times a day. It is a social experience and although dining settings vary enormously, the real value of mealtime rests in the interpersonal exchange it provides. Mealtime in an institution for the frail elderly *can* be a dining experience that not only stimulates appetite and aids digestion but also creates a social milieu. But in order to facilitate good eating experiences in an institution for the frail elderly there must be certain essential ingredients: a pleasant, designated dining space, adequate furniture and other equipment which fits diners needs and enables them to manage eating activities, and helping personnel with specific knowledge, skills and attitudes to provide assistance.

This paper will describe some of the factors that contribute to successful dining experiences in institutions for frail and sick elderly persons and examine the role for occupational therapy in those environments.

ESTABLISHING A DINING PROGRAM

Elderly persons need and want the same things that others expect within their dining environments. For instance, what things do you like when dining away from home? What is it like to eat alone if you have always eaten with others? What is your reaction if there is a lot of noise and confusion created by a rushed environment? Does the food served look appealing, and smell and taste good? Are there any decorations or features of the setting which make the mood pleasant? These same things should be factors to consider in dining settings in institutions, as well as other ingredients which contribute to the eating experience being both successful and satisfying to residents.

The purpose of a 'dining program' within an institution is to provide the structure needed to make an environment as 'normal' as possible, so as to promote 'best' skill levels, insure consistent approaches to residents from staff, in a setting that allows management and organization of the dining space to afford both good service and socialization among *all* present. A well arranged and managed dining space promotes efficiency for staff and the well-being of residents because it creates the environment in which residents can eat and staff can provide both appropriate help and the incentives for social interaction. Successful dining goes beyond tablecloths and centerpieces. The social climate in a dining room is created not just by its physical characteristics but by the general atmosphere, overall appearance, background sounds, how residents are seated and the way equipment and tools for eating are used. Personnel are keys to the tone within the setting as they establish the tempo of activity and set the environmental mood.

In establishing a program there must first be a 'space' that is designated as a dining area, or an area that can be easily transformed into a dining room at mealtimes. Any space can be made more pleasant by color, lighting, decoration as well as arrangement of furniture to create social groups and still make resident and staff mobility easy. For the frail elderly the size of furniture and its accessibility is critical. Wheelchairs when needed must be able to fit under table tops and must afford adequate posture for the activities of eating. (Postural supports and cushions, footrests adjusted to correct position to afford foot pressure to help the occupant stay upright are often needed.) Regular dining chairs when used should have arms to help support the person when seated and to offer a push-off when the person is rising or transferring. The setting, in other words, should foster independence and social interaction at highest levels rather than sullen and silent dependency.

It is in creating such positive environments that the skills and philosophy of an occupational therapist can be vital in assisting staff to develop such settings that encourage each resident to function at his/her highest. This involves grouping residents with like cognitive abilities to encourage interchange as well as providing supports/equipment to accommodate any physical limitations residents may have that interfere with independent eating. Thus a 'normalized' environment can be a part of every institutional dining setting thereby offering one basic motivation for eating.

Residents With Special Needs

Residents whose independence in eating is deteriorating or whose abilities to relate with others is hampered by sensory losses should be evaluated by the occupational therapist to see if problems are physical or mental or both. Typical physical problems related to eating are inability to complete hand to mouth movements, problems presented by the excursion distance (average distance should be 10–12 inches), poor or unstable sitting posture, visual difficulties, general weakness or low endurance. In addition persons may have oral motor problems (chewing, swallowing). This is a whole separate area of need which will not be addressed in this paper, but is a logical concern of the occupational therapist working together with nursing personnel.

In addition, it is not uncommon that elderly persons are confused by any new or different environment (from their bed living space) and may need cues to carry out even simple eating activities because of the distractions around them. The results of such problems are clear. For the resident, dining is an unpleasant experience. Food spills, utensils cannot be handled adequately, a great deal of energy may be unnecessarily expended as the person struggles to get food—providing he is interested. More likely, as frustration increases from lack of satisfactory eating, interest in food wanes and the benefit of being with others is lost in the difficulties being encountered. Finally nutrition suffers, the person is fed by others (many times to his embarrassment and distaste) and a vicious cycle begins.

For the occupational therapist consulting in such settings the tendency is to concentrate solely on the specific eating problems individuals have rather than on the total environment and management of eating and mealtime procedures. Obviously one should work on both aspects of the situation in order to institute a satisfactory *dining* program. Since residents in facilities for the frail elderly vary considerably in both physical and mental abilities, each one must be evaluated as an individual as one begins to make dining a positive experience.

Creating a Homelike Atmosphere

An institution can reflect a family atmosphere, especially in the dining room. The social level of the dining room will determine the types of interaction that result. Naturally, residents who can initiate conversation and respond to social environments **require different** relationships from staff than those residents who **require** sensory stimulation and re-motivation activities. An institutional dining room may represent every level of cognitive ability and thus must be arranged to accommodate all those differences. It is therefore necessary first to establish 'social levels' among the residents, and do 'social' groupings for eating activities. This may even be best done in multiple dining areas, even though within every level of cognitive or social ability there may be persons with highest to lowest levels of physical independence in eating. Staff must be assigned to accommodate both social and physical needs of diners, but residents are placed in groups *first* according to social level, then by physical skill level. In any case, for those residents who still can and do enjoy social interaction, the dining plans in an institution should offer that opportunity first and foremost, since meal times are the major times of the day in which socialization with friends can occur. More will be said about arrangements of groups later.

Just as the grouping of residents affords interaction, there must be the atmosphere in the setting that stimulates exchange. Decorations in the room for those who can enjoy same, table arrangements, lighting, attention to noise levels to afford conversation, participation by staff in helping those who require physical help done in as unobtrusive ways as possible, preferably seated next to the person being helped and taking part in the social group. The *behaviors* of families should be encouraged if family atmospheres are to be created.

Accommodating Physical/Mechanical Needs

In whatever seating the resident uses for eating, *positioning* is the first concern of the occupational therapist. Chairs should provide for posture in which hips, knees and ankles are stabilized and supported at 90 degrees, since that is the posture required for normal 'at table' eating. If any deformity is noted that interferes with functional posture, changes in seating, table or techniques of eating should be instituted.

Regular Chairs

In general, regular chairs for dining areas should be chosen with the following features:

1. An arm chair with a 16-inch-high *seat* slightly padded and slightly inclined at the front both for comfort and to prevent sliding forward. Seats should be not too wide or deep as older persons in general are of small stature. Feet should touch the floor.
2. Chairs should be *stable*, with a firm base, not easily tipped during transfers.
3. *Arms* should extend just three-fourths of the seat depth to allow the chair to fit under a regular height table and be wide enough to provide good grip surface while the person rises or transfers.
4. *Design* should be simple, construction material such that repairs can be made when necessary and all surfaces can be easily cleaned. Chairs should be sturdy enough to withstand the ordinary battering of heavy use and collision with wheelchairs.
5. Any regular chair used should also be such that seat belts or security ties can be used if needed for safety. Unfortunately many institutions use personal jacket-type restraints for this purpose. Many residents find them too restrictive and object to such constraints on personal freedom.

Wheelchairs

For residents who eat while in wheelchairs the following conditions should be met. Here also the occupational therapist is the staff person who can most logically supervise choice and fit of wheelchairs.

1. Chairs should *fit* the resident—width, depth of seat; height of back; distance to foot rests.
2. *Seats* should be made firm and level by using posture cushions or other supports to assure stable posture. There are a number of posture cushions available. Bed pillows do not serve well for sitting surfaces.
3. Since *arm rests* are necessary for support, they should be of desk type so that the chair can fit under regular tables.
4. There should be workable *locks*, and *seat belts*, if needed. A person eating in a wheelchair needs to be in a stable, secure position.
5. *Lap trays* should be available in order to allow residents to be

a part of a social group if chair does not fit under tables used. Surfaces should be light colored, unmarred and easily kept clean.

Tables

A dining area generally will have tables of standard height (28–30″) both to accommodate ambulatory residents or those transferred to regular chairs for eating. Also if wheelchairs have cut-away arms, persons using them will have access to regular tables. Round tables can be more flexible for grouping residents and are thought by some to be also more attractive and functional. Staff find with round tables better space for assisting those who require physical help, and better socialization results if small groupings (4–6) are used. Sensory deficits (hearing, vision) otherwise could limit conversation and exchange. For those residents who require special assistance and/or equipment lap tables may prove more efficient to use (less spillage) and chairs can still be arranged so that conversations and interrelating is possible. Good lighting to table tops is essential.

Table surface-to-mouth excursion distance is critical to success in eating for many persons with eating problems cited earlier. Normal plate to mouth distance for adults is 10–12 inches. For eating liquids, juicy or unstable foods the distance must be shorter (8–10″). Therefore, depending on the innate ability of the person, these distances may need to be altered or eating style accommodated to make eating activity successful. Occupational therapists are accustomed to adapting either the *method*, the *setting* or the *equipment used* in an activity to promote independence. Accordingly, some accommodations will be required if residents are uncoordinated, have diminished strength or endurance, need special eating equipment (scoop dishes, swivel or built-up utensils, non-spill cups, etc.). If persons have limited range of motion in upper extremities additional positioning or equipment adaptations will be required. Nothing is more personally defeating or embarrassing than spilling or obvious awkwardness in eating while with others. Further, if one must concentrate all attention on mechanical aspects of eating, the social part of the mealtime will surely be lost.

In summary, by providing residents with secure and comfortable seating, the ability to see, smell and reach their food, the first step in creating a *dining environment* has been taken. For now each resident, according to his own interests and level of cognitive ability, can focus attention and effort not just to eating activities but to being a part of the social environment of the setting.

STAFF ROLES IN CREATING DINING PROGRAMS

Just as at home, eating in an institution can be enhanced by conversation, shared participation and stimulation of senses. While at home or eating with friends when dining out one creates a family atmosphere in the process. One's habits and values influence how one behaves. Similarly in institutions a family atmosphere can be created—by the setting, by staff attitudes and expectations and behaviors, by modeling the kinds of interaction they wish to support.

Some of the *personnel* characteristics of a successful dining program are as follows:

1. An agreed upon philosophy in the facility to create a home-like environment and one individual with responsibility and authority to see it is carried out. This includes seeing that all residents possible get to the dining room for each group meal.
2. Specific evaluation of eating skills of each resident as a routine procedure so that individual 'eating assistance regimes' can be established and rechecked regularly.
3. Enough information and instruction as necessary for all staff to assure that each resident's needs and preferences in eating are known.
4. Availability of adequate staff to provide assistance during meal hours, and to be a part of the social groups to provide extra stimulation and support for socialization and independent functioning.
5. Some leader from among facility staff to assure that the 'things' that help to create dining environments are provided—decorations, favors, diets fitted to residents needs and special occasions, food kept attractive, some plan for interaction among those who can participate at every meal. This is frequently made viable by work with volunteers, advocates, ombudsmen.
6. Above all a caring attitude that encourages residents to stay

active and as independent as possible and allows choices whenever possible.

An occupational therapist with comprehensive concerns for quality of life in institutions for the frail elderly can be the stimulus to the development and implementation of successful dining programs as well as for the preservation of individual rights in settings where dependency is often a hallmark of residing there. The therapist who creates good relationships with staff counterparts—the administrator, the charge nurse, the dietitian, the maintenance supervisor as well as with daily service personnel—can demonstrate ways in which a dining program that respects individual preferences and needs, and is dedicated to providing family style social groups in which each resident can participate according to his/her level, will be efficient and effective. It will require less rather than more work in the long run and above all, residents will be experiencing a better quality of daily living, with dignity, surrounded by a caring, helpful staff. Carry-over to other aspects of daily routines is also made easier with such fundamental attitudes prevailing.

SUMMARY AND CONCLUSIONS

The elements involved in creating dining programs in institutions for the frail elderly have been described and discussed along with the role of the occupational therapist as the catalyst in implementing such programs. The importance of evaluating individual resident's needs and creating dining groups according to 'social levels,' and thus enhancing potentials for participation in a family-like environment was emphasized. Some specific criteria for choosing and arranging the setting for dining was also discussed. However, emphasis was given to the importance of staff, and staff attitudes, as the keys to success of any successful dining program.

The atmosphere and appearance of a dining room enhances the eating environment. A dining room can be a beautifully designed space or a solarium that becomes the dining room, but it is not the actual room that is important. Rather, it is what is done to the room so that it becomes a *dining* room that stimulates the dining experience. With creative thinking and good problem solving, simple measures such as using centerpieces, placemats, appetizers, plate service, waitress service, staff sitting down when they assist

residents, music, controlled background noise, good conversation—
all these create overall atmosphere and appearance that defines the
expectations of both function and service within the room. In a
sense they define for the resident and staff what their expected
behaviors should be. These elements of dining strategy coupled with
socialization and the physical ability to eat can make dining within
a health care setting a pleasurable experience for staff and residents
alike.

SUGGESTED READINGS

Beck C: Dining experiences of the institutionalized aged. *J Ger Nurs* 7(2) 1981
Bergen A: Positioning the Client with Central Nervous System Deficits: The Wheelchair and
    Other Adapted Equipment. Valhalla Rehabilitation Publications, 1983
Clancy K L: Preliminary observations on media use and food habits of the elderly.
    Gerontologist 15(6) 529–532, 1975
Keebler N: Nutrition: A social factor. *Contemp Admin* 5:10–13, 1979
Mandal A C: The seated man: The seated work position. Theory and practice. *Appl Ergon* 3:
    19–25, 1981
Savitsky E and Zetterstrom M: Group feeding for the elderly. *J Am Diet Assoc* 35: 938, 1959
Sherwood S: Sociology of food and eating: Implications for action for the elderly. *Am J Clin
    Nutr* 26:1108–1110, 1973
Sherwood S and Krause E: A dining room behavior study. Paper presented at the Eighth
    International Congress of Gerontology, Washington, D.C., August 1969
Perket S, Drews J, et al.: Back to the Table: A Practical Approach to Long Term Care Dining
    Programs. Edina, MN: St Croix Therapy, Inc., 1984
St. Croix Therapy: A Motivational Dining Study, 1983. Unpublished paper
Valenti, Vincent: Back to the Table: Identification and Solutions of Problems in Institutional
    Feeding Programs for the Aged. Multimedia presentation. St. Croix Therapy, Inc., 1982
Weg R B: Nutrition and the Later Years

REFERENCE

1. Beck C, as above

Swallowing Problems in Patients With Head and Neck Cancer: The Role of Occupational Therapy

Christine B. Jensen, MS, OTR
David L. Evans, RN, MSN

ABSTRACT. The restoration of swallowing skills in head and neck cancer surgery patients demands a two-pronged approach: thorough and systematic evaluation and simple, fundamental treatments. Therapists should begin with an assessment of their own biases and their knowledge of head and neck cancer and its surgeries. The patients themselves should be evaluated both presurgically—to determine food preferences, other medical conditions, nutritional status, and current swallowing abilities, and postsurgically—to assess facial symmetry, oral mobility and strength, saliva management, aspiration risk, and altered swallowing skills. Treatment approaches should generally be basic, stressing oral exercises, positioning techniques, the use of feeding aids, and teaching the supraglottic swallow. Attention to certain special considerations, like problems with cuffed tracheostomies and the controversies over using variable food consistencies, will refine the treatment.

While head and neck cancer comprises just 5% of all cancer in the United States, its effect on the individual can be devastating. To attack the cancer, the mouth, throat, and vocal cords are surgically resected, the neck dissected, with the head and neck subjected to subsequent radiation as well. Their cancer at least momentarily expunged, the patients' initial relief is soon followed by anger, withdrawal, embarrassment, and frustration. New problems emerge. Their faces are hideously disfigured. If they can talk at all, their voices gurgle and crack. They may drool, sputter, and cough

Christine B. Jensen is an occupational therapist and David L. Evans is a nurse practitioner at Oklahoma Children's Memorial Hospital, Oklahoma City, OK.

This article appears jointly in *Occupational Therapy for People With Eating Dysfunctions* (The Haworth Press, Inc., 1986) and *Occupational Therapy in Health Care*, Volume 3, Number 2 (Summer 1986).

when they eat. Some fear choking to death. The most basic elements of human development—breathing, swallowing, and eating—often become heroic efforts.

Occupational therapists may be duly hesitant to tackle these difficulties, but they are in a special position to do so. Because of their training in psychosocial as well as physical dysfunction and because they emphasize restoring function in even the most basic tasks of daily life, such as eating, the occupational therapist is specially qualified to help these cancer patients surmount their problems.

This paper outlines how the therapist might contribute to the basic restoration of eating and swallowing skills in head and neck cancer patients, including suggestions on how to systematically assess such patients and describing some basic therapeutic techniques.

EVALUATION OF ONESELF

Helping the head and neck cancer patient should begin with an honest assessment of the therapist's own biases and knowledge. The therapist may feel, for example, that the patient brought the problem on himself. Indeed, many have long histories of tobacco and alcohol abuse contributing to their disease. Many are not able or willing to change their lifestyles after surgery. Moreover, the therapist who has not confronted her own expectations may find the patient physically repugnant. Faces are sometimes rearranged and swollen, tubes dangling everywhere, tracheostomies and stomas draining foul-smelling mucus. Because the patients themselves are often repulsed by their altered bodies, they are particularly sensitive to the responses of those around them, including the occupational therapist.

Just as importantly, the therapist should assess her expectations for progress, knowing that it may be like a roller coaster, small gains coupled with severe setbacks. After weeks of struggling with something as simple as a workable swallow, the therapist may be met with a recurrence of the cancer itself or even the patient's imminent death.

Finally, assuming the therapist feels she can work with this group of people, she should also assess her knowledge of normal swallowing and of the surgical procedures involved with head and neck cancer, both generally and those specifically done on her patient. Useful reviews of normal swallowing[1-4] and general surgery of the head and neck[5,6] are available. The therapist will need specifically to learn the size and location of the tumor and the extent of the surgery and reconstruction, since these variations in surgical procedures and lesions can greatly affect swallowing. For example, during a floor of mouth excision, the defect may be filled either with the tongue, which results in significant eating problems, or with a flap of tissue from some other body part, which results in minimal eating problems.

EVALUATION OF THE PATIENT

Armed with an assessment of herself, the therapist is ready to evaluate the patient himself, both presurgically and postsurgically.

Presurgical Assessment. Ideally, the therapist should see the patient prior to surgery. Because of the trauma of surgery and because many patients rely heavily on oral communication skills rather than writing skills, it is much more difficult to obtain adequate information after surgery. Presurgically, the therapist can determine if the patient is currently having problems eating and swallowing. Some patients report just a loss of appetite, while others report that, because of the nature of the tumor, it is just too painful to eat or swallow. Some have had radiation therapy, which may either make their mouths very dry, or cause their saliva to become thick and copious. Also, many patients have had significant weight loss prior to hospitalization. Since good nutritional status is important to successful healing, the therapist may need to work closely with the physician and dietician to be sure the patient gets enough calories. If he is having difficulty swallowing liquid, then perhaps soft foods and thicker liquids, such as malts, will help. If he is having trouble chewing and eating regular foods, then more concentrated liquids, such as instant breakfasts, or complete liquid formulas such as Ensure, or Isocal, will help.

The presurgical period is also a good time to assess current eating habits and preferences and other medical conditions that may affect food choices after surgery. Such a simple task as discovering a patient's favorite or least favorite foods may be vitally important. For example, a cancer patient on our service once was assumed to have a special swallowing disorder when he refused to eat his clear liquid diet. It was found, however, that he could swallow well but simply hated the Jellos and broths making up much of his daily meals. After the physicians were convinced to advance his diet to purees and he was able to eat mashed potatoes and creamed soups, his intake improved considerably. A presurgical assessment could have eliminated this misunderstanding from the start. Additionally, broader cultural preferences should be noted; for example, the milk product base for some of the soft foods selected may be unpalatable in some ethnic cultures. Finally, medical conditions such as diabetes or hypercholesterolemia may be important in deciding what foods to use after surgery.

Gathering all this information suggests that these patients will definitely have difficulty swallowing after surgery. But the therapist should not assume this and should not warn the patients ahead of time. Giving them one more thing to worry about before surgery is generally not helpful. Many patients, in fact, are quite resilient and resourceful and do quite well. The therapist should just let them know that *if* they should have any problems, she will be there to help, letting such reassurance be the base for the rapport needed to work with them afterward.

Postsurgical Assessment. After surgery, the therapist should be prepared for a considerable wait before finishing the evaluation of the patient and beginning therapy. If any eating or swallowing structures were involved during surgery, it is usually 10–14 days before patients are started on oral feedings and then only on clear liquids. Although liquids are more difficult to manage and control and there is greater risk of aspirating liquids, physicians feel the incidence of infection is less with liquids, and such foods place less stress on recently operated sites.

Until patients are able to swallow sufficient calories, they are maintained on nasogastric tube feedings. Occasionally, some patients will complain that the tube makes swallowing uncomfortable, so some therapists suggest removing the tube for feeding sessions. However, most patients find that having the tube replaced after each feeding session creates more discomfort than swallowing with it in place. The therapist will need to work with the patient in determining what option is best.

Specifically, the postsurgical evaluation should assess general facial symmetry, mobility and strength of the tongue, mouth, and jaw, management of saliva, including the likelihood of aspiration, and ability to swallow. First, *facial symmetry* should be observed for any signs of paralysis. Second, to take food off a spoon and keep it in the mouth, the lips need a certain amount of *mobility*. The patient may no longer be able to fully purse, open and close, or retract the lips, all limitations that should be noted. Third, *tongue mobility* is crucial to forming food into a bolus and transporting it from the front of the mouth to the back of the throat. The therapist should check the patient's ability to protrude the tongue beyond the lips, move it laterally, touch the roof of the mouth, and retract or "hump" the tongue. Fourth, since sufficient *jaw opening* is necessary to admit food to the mouth and to permit good oral hygiene, the therapist should observe the patient's ability to open the jaw wide and move it from side to side. Surgical manipulation of the jaw (mandibular splits and swings) or resection (marginal or segmental) may have caused sufficient trauma to the temporo-mandibular joint to make these maneuvers very difficult.

Fifth, the therapist should observe how well the patient can *manage his saliva* and secretions and what his risk of *aspiration* is likely to be. If he is not swallowing his saliva, she should determine why. Some patients, for example, report their saliva is initially too objectionable and do not want to swallow it. Others report it will not go down or it hurts to swallow, while others have problems managing it because of poor lip closure, causing drooling.

An assessment of a patient's saliva management should be closely linked with an evaluation of aspiration. The medical literature does not indicate how much aspiration is acceptable, though some doctors believe any is too much. However, most head and neck surgeons feel comfortable with a slight amount of aspiration if the patient has a good protective cough and this minimal aspiration is believed to be a temporary problem. The individual therapist should determine both the physician's tolerance here and her own. Still, since aspiraton is at worst life-threatening and at best an important factor in swallowing and eating progress, the therapist should learn to evaluate it. Assuming they are not the result of radiation therapy, copious, thick, or tenacious oral secretions may be a sign of aspiration, although the therapist may get more useful clinical information by noting the quality of voice. If the patient has a tracheostomy, the therapist should occlude it to hear his voice. If it sounds gargly or raspy, it could mean he is aspirating, with secretions, saliva, and food resting in the larynx above the vocal cords. In such cases, the therapist can have the patient clear his throat or cough to clear any particles from the larynx and see if the voice improves. If the patient cannot cough here, later safe swallowing will be difficult and should be postponed until he can.

Unfortunately, some of these patients may be "silent aspirators,"[4] aspiration occurring even as the food goes down without any coughing or choking. Thus, the therapist should always observe other signs, like temperature increases, that may indicate aspiration pneumonia. Because minimizing aspiraton is so vital to the patient's progress, she should not hesitate to encourage the physician to order a cine esophogram or videofluoroscopy if she feels aspiration is present and is not being detected by others.

Finally, the therapist can assess *swallowing skills* post-surgically even though this may not be possible until 10–14 days after surgery when the patient begins eating. In a quiet environment, the therapist should talk with the patient about the swallowing trial, letting him know what she is looking for and asking him to concentrate as well, so he can tell her exactly where a problem originates. If necessary, nursing personnel can suction the patient's mouth, tracheostomy, or stoma, so the patient can begin with a "clean" mouth. The patient can then take a tiny sip of water (or the therapist can use a straw as a pipette to introduce 1/3 tsp. water, or use ice chips) in the mouth and ask the patient to swallow it. The therapist should watch carefully to see if it is transported normally to the back of the throat. If the water slips forward and drools out, the patient may have oral cavity problems, including problems with lip closure or lack of tongue mobility. If he coughs and chokes *before* he swallows, this also indicates an oral cavity problem where the liquid is spilling into the pharynx before it is controlled. If he chokes *during* the swallow, the larynx is not elevating and closing off during the swallow. If he chokes *after* the swallow, some residue liquid is left in the pharynx (specifically in the valleculae or pyriform sinuses) after the swallow and then spills over into the larynx. After the swallow, the therapist should check for any residue left in the mouth and then check the patient's voice quality to see if any residue may be resting in the larynx. Some therapists add food color to the liquid so that if material coughed out of the trach/stoma site or suctioned from the larynx is colored, then they know the patient has aspirated some and can estimate how much.

In summary, a thorough and systematic assessment of the patient before and after surgery, prior to any therapeutic intervention, will yield valuable baseline information on the idiosyncrasies of the patient and on the nature and extent of his particular difficulty. Such data encourage more individual and realistic treatment.

TREATMENT

Although treatment approaches vary, the Oklahoma Teaching Hospital has found the following four emphases to be useful. Characteristically stressed are oral exercises, positioning techniques, the use of feeding aids, and teaching the supraglottic swallow and other swallowing exercises.

I. Oral Exercises

Most of the problems in eating and swallowing are caused by structural and physical alterations to the lip, tongue, or jaw during surgery, unlike the neurological deficits seen with stroke patients, though some patients can have both types. Oral exercises are particularly useful in reducing these physical limitations if they are done consistently for one to two months after surgery.

To improve lip closure, tongue blades are stacked together the width of the lip opening and patients are asked to squeeze with their lips, holding this position for one second and progressively increasing the hold to one minute. Gradually the number of tongue blades is decreased until he can hold one firmly for one minute. Lip closure will also be aided by facial expression exercises—pursing and retracting the lips and baring the teeth— much as one does for patients with neurological deficits of the face.

To increase tongue mobility, range of motion exercises such as protruding, retracting, elevating, and moving the tongue from side to side are used. To increase tongue strength, these same exercises can be done while providing resistance with a tongue blade. For fine tongue control, a rolled up square of gauze (with a string attached for safety) or a licorice whip, is placed on the roof of the mouth, and the patient is asked to hold it there with his tongue to encourage the tongue to shape and hold a bolus. If, after these exercises, the tongue still cannot reach the roof of the mouth, oral exercises may be inadequate and an intraoral prosthesis may be needed. For even finer tongue control, the patient is asked to move a small object, like a Life Saver attached to a string, from one side of the mouth to the other (i.e., the lateral sulcus).[4]

To increase mobility in stiff and painful jaws after surgery, range of motion exercises are used, including opening the mouth as wide as the patient can and holding that position for a set time, moving the jaw from side to side, and making circles with the jaw.

II. Positioning

Positioning the head during swallowing may be used as a compensatory technique until the patient regains oropharyngeal control or as a permanent way to assist swallowing. These techniques do *not*, however, change the physiology of swallowing but simply assist gravity in controlling the flow of food.

Many therapists recommend a single posture for optimal safe swallowing—sitting upright with the head flexed forward—but not all patients swallow better in this position. If lip closure is a problem or tongue mobility is poor, then tilting the head back when swallowing is more helpful. If the patient has had a total glossectomy, he often does better with the "gulp" or "dump and swallow" technique, during which the patient holds the head back and continues swallowing. Since the patient will aspirate small amounts during this technique, he should be encouraged to cough periodically.

If the deficit is in the pharynx, lateral head positions may be more successful in aiding swallowing and preventing aspiration, since the problem here is usually unilateral. If, for example, the right side of the pharynx is impaired and the patient is having problems with aspiration after the swallow, then *rotating* the head to the right will close off the right pyriform sinus and allow food to go down the left side. This prevents food from collecting in the right pyriform sinus and possibly spilling over into the larynx after a swallow. Likewise, the same effect may be achieved by *tilting* the head to the left, thus allowing gravity to direct food down the left side of the pharynx.

If the problem is in the larynx, then flexing the head forward before swallowing will usually allow the tongue to fall down and the epiglottis to fold over, protecting the airway. When the damage is to one vocal cord, rotating the head to the involved side puts pressure on that vocal cord, thus increasing its adduction and minimizing aspiration during swallowing.

III. Feeding Aids

Although often fearful of choking or embarrassing themselves, most head and neck cancer patients are still eager to eat and rid themselves of their feeding tubes. Many, in fact, attempt to eat and swallow before they are completely healed. Special feeding aids are thus needed with this group.

Unfortunately, the most widely promoted aid—the glossectomy spoon or "pusher" spoon—is probably the least effective. This spoon is designed to push food off into the back of the throat. However, patients in our service could not position the spoon correctly in their mouths, mostly because of problems with decreased or altered sensation. The spoon has also been too big for most patients' mouths. Further, it has not always done a good job of pushing the food off where desired either. If solid or soft foods need to be placed in the back of the throat, most patients have felt more comfortable with regular spoons.

Generally, however, most patients are begun on liquids and have poor lip closure or tongue control. Such patients are unable to use spoons of any kind at first. Two aids have proven useful for these patients. A 50cc Toomy syringe with a French #14 catheter cut to appropriate length, enables some patients to drink liquids with very little spilling (Figure 1). Still, this is often just a temporary measure, since most patients want to eat normally as quickly as possible. The special "nosey" cup promotes this. The device, a simple cup with a deep arc cut into one side, allows the patient to drink normally without having to tilt the head markedly (Figure 2). Eventually, many patients will advance beyond this and drink with a regular cup, tilting the head back to decrease drooling, even though they may still rely heavily on Ensure, Isocal, high calorie malts, or thinned purees. It is tempting to minimize the importance of such simple devices, but they serve a vital role in freeing the patient from a feeding tube, fostering independence and restoring a more normal appearance.

IV. Supraglottic Swallow and Swallowing Exercises

Three structures protect the airway from food during swallowing: (1) the epiglottis and aryepiglottic fold; (2) the false vocal cords; and (3) the true vocal cords. Tumors in the supraglottic region usually necessitate a supraglottic laryngectomy in which the first two

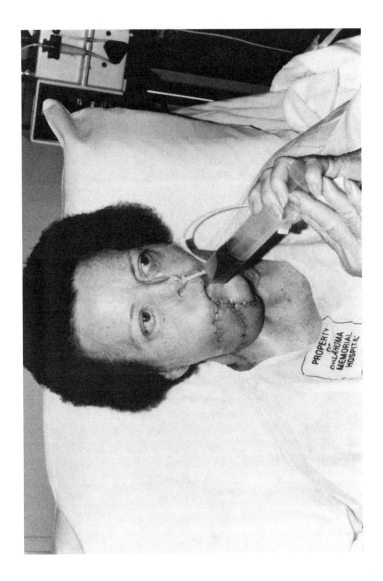

FIGURE 1. Use of Toomy syringe with catheter attached for patient with poor lip closure and poor tongue mobility.

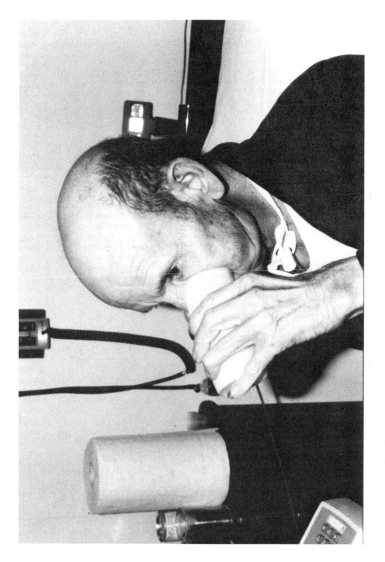

FIGURE 2. Use of "nosey" cup for patient with no tongue mobility and inability to tip head back.

protective structures are removed, leaving only the two true vocal cords to shield the airway.

To further protect the airway against aspiration, patients in this group can be taught the supraglottic swallow, or the swallow-cough-swallow technique. The patient is instructed to hold his breath (or occlude his tracheostomy), swallow, cough, swallow again, and then breathe. Holding the breath causes the true vocal cords to adduct, thus preventing food from passing into the airway. Since some particles may fall and rest on the vocal cords, coughing and swallowing again will "blow" any residue off. If the patient inhales before coughing, the residue will be sucked into the airway.

The technique above will be helpful for any patient with true vocal cords that will adduct but without the other two protective structures. If vocal cord adduction is not complete, adduction exercises will help. For example, while seated and holding his breath, (or occluding the tracheostoma) the patient pulls firmly on the sides of the chair seat—much like a valsalva maneuver—for five seconds. This exercise is then repeated with only one hand while the patient says "ah" long, clear, and continuously. Finally, the patient, still holding onto the chair seat with one hand, says "ah" five times in quick succession.[4]

Patients who have had a hemilaryngectomy or vertical laryngectomy probably will not need this technique, since the epiglottis remains and the false and true vocal cord can still adduct against remaining scar tissue. If they do experience problems with aspiration, tipping the head forward should give them sufficient airway protection during swallowing.

The therapies suggested in sections I-IV above assume an optimistic prognoses for the patient. Unfortunately, not all of these patients will become functional eaters. If after working on positioning techniques, special feedings aids, or on swallowing exercises, the patient is still unable to take in sufficient calories or is unsatisfied with the selected swallowing method, longterm nasogastric tube feedings or gastrostomy tube feedings will need to be considered.

SPECIAL CONSIDERATIONS

Independent of other swallowing evaluations or techniques, two special considerations may affect the patient's progress—tracheostomies and food consistencies. Tracheostomy tubes are present in many head and neck cancer patients to assure an adequate airway. Generally, patients are fitted with a cuffed trach for the first 4–5 days postoperatively or until they can manage their secretions either by swallowing them or by suctioning them orally. This is then replaced as soon as possible with a noncuffed trach to reduce laryngeal irritation. Swallowing is thus usually started with a noncuffed trach. The therapist will need to proceed cautiously in the beginning, using very small amounts of water or food, being sure the patient has an adequate cough, and having nursing personnel available for suctioning if necessary. If, on the other hand, the patient has a cuffed trach, it should remain deflated during swallowing trials. This prevents laryngeal erosion and allows the therapist to determine when aspiration occurs if the patient begins to choke or cough. For example, if food or water is allowed to pile up over an inflated cuff, the therapist will know aspiration occurred only after deflating the cuff and will not be able to evaluate the precise cause of the problem.

Inattention to food consistencies can also delay progress. Generally, patients with poor oral control and reduced pharyngeal peristalsis will do better with liquids. However, patients with reduced laryngeal closure or delayed swallow reflex will do better with thicker foods. Therapists, too, will differ in their recommendations for the same patient, some using carbonated liquids, others not. Some recommend cold or warm foods and others will not. In the end, the important thing to remember is that one food, consistency, or temperature will not work for every patient. Attention to the individual patient, a knowledge of the cancer and the surgery, and some safe trial and error will usually dictate what is best.

CONCLUSION

When occupational therapists work with swallowing and eating disorders among head and neck cancer patients, they are often too anxious to treat. They sometimes forget that a thorough assessment of both the patient's peculiar situation and the therapist's own biases and knowledge ought to precede any intervention. When they do begin treatment, the therapists are often too eager to forge complex and ambitious plans, forgetting that the most apparently simple treatments, like oral and swallowing exercises and basic positioning techniques, may be the most elegant and effective ways to restore dignity and function as these patients learn anew to swallow and eat.

REFERENCES

1. Aguilar NV, Olsen ML, Shedd DP: Deglutition problems in patients with head and neck cancer. *Am J Surg* 138(4):501–507, 1979

2. Dobie RA: Rehabilitation of swallowing disorders. *Am Fam Phys* 17(5):84–95, 1978

3. Conley JC: Swallowing dysfunction associated with radical surgery of the head and neck. *Arch Surg* 80:602–612, 1960

4. Logemann JA: Evaluation and Treatment of Swallowing Disorders. San Diego: College-Hill Press, 1983

5. Lore JM: An Atlas of Head and Neck Surgery, 2nd Ed., Vol. II. Philadelphia: Saunders Co., 1973

6. Naumann HH: Head and Neck Surgery, Vol. II. Philadelphia: Saunders Co., 1980

BIBLIOGRAPHY

Conley JC: *Complications of Head and Neck Surgery*. Philadelphia: Saunders Co., 1979

Dudgeon BJ, DeLisa JA, Miller RM: Head and neck cancer, a rehabilitation approach. *Am J Occup Ther* 34(4)243–251, 1980

Logemann JA, Bytell DE: Swallowing disorders in three types of head and neck surgical patients. *Cancer* 44(3)1095–1105, 1979

Sessions DG, Zill R, Schwartz SL: Deglutition after conservation surgery for cancer of the larynx and hypopharynx *Otolaryngol Head Neck Surg* 87:779–796, 1979

Trible WM: The rehabilitation of deglutition following head and neck surgery. *Laryngol* 77:518–523, 1967

Weaver AW, Fleming SM: Partial laryngectomy: Analysis of associated swallowing disorders. *Am J Surg* 136:486–489, 1978

Oral Motor and Feeding Problems in the Tube Fed Infant: Suggested Treatment Strategies for the Occupational Therapist

Susan Vogel, MHS, OTR

ABSTRACT. Relatively little information has been available to prepare occupational therapists to meet the special needs of the tube fed infant. The purpose of this paper is to share specific information through a literature review regarding oral motor and feeding intervention for the tube fed infant who also may have a tracheostomy. Suggested treatment strategies are also discussed and illustrated in a case example.

Infants with neurological deficits often display oral motor problems, such as incoordination of suck, swallow and breathing, inefficient suck-swallow, and orofacial hypersensitivity.[1] These problems may lead to inefficient feeding with poor food intake, limited bonding between infant and parent, and later difficulties in independent self feeding.[2] Occupational therapists often work with the neurologically impaired infant to improve oral motor and feeding skills. Basic professional and continuing education in oral motor intervention for the neurologically impaired infant have qualified many occupational therapists to meet the special self care needs of this population. It seems there have been less educational opportunities, however, for occupational therapists to develop the specialized skills necessary to meet the unique needs of the neurologically impaired infant who receives enteral nutritional

Susan Vogel is an assistant professor, Occupational Therapy Program, Cleveland State University, Cleveland, OH. She also has a small private practice serving pediatric clients.

The author gratefully acknowledges the editorial assistance of John Bazyk, MS, OTR.

This article appears jointly in *Occupational Therapy for People With Eating Dysfunctions* (The Haworth Press, Inc., 1986) and *Occupational Therapy in Health Care*, Volume 3, Number 2 (Summer 1986).

63

support via tube feedings. The purpose of this article is to review the literature on the tube fed infant and the infant with tracheostomy and to discuss treatment implications for this population based on the literature review and author's clinical experience.

The specific population addressed in this article is the neurologically impaired infant who is fed by nasogastric tube (NG tube) or gastrostomy tube (G tube), and who may have a tracheostomy. Often enteral nutritional support via tube feedings is initiated in infants with severe swallowing problems, causing difficult and lengthy feeding sessions, nutritional deprivation, aspiration, and chronic lung disease.[3] Enteral nutritional support (food entering stomach or intestines) is generally the intervention of choice over parenteral methods (nourishment received outside intestines e.g., intravenous) because it is viewed as more economical and effective in maintaining or improving the nutrition of non-oral feeders.[4,5] Generally, if non-oral feedings are anticipated to be temporary (lasting less than 3 months) then NG tube feeding is the treatment of choice.[6] The gastrostomy is a surgical procedure that is preferred when non-oral feedings are predicted to be long-term (more than 3 months).[6] Tracheostomy placement is often indicated in patients with severe airway problems that result in the need for prolonged ventilation.[7] During the past two decades indications for airway management via tracheostomy have broadened because of an increased survival rate among infants treated for prematurity and for congenital cardiac and foregut anomalies.[7]

As an occupational therapist working with infants with the above described conditions, the author began to observe some behaviors during oral feeding sessions that seemed different from infants experiencing oral motor difficulties as a result of neurological deficits alone. Some of the behaviors include (a) inconsistencies in oral hypersensitivity, for example enjoyment of self-induced mouthing of toys and objects, but crying and gagging when the feeder approached the mouth with a finger of food; (b) the appearance of purposeful avoidance of swallowing food by sustained jaw extension and tongue retraction; (c) the presence of avoidance behaviors during feeding, such as turning the head away from food, pushing away the food, and falling asleep during the session, and (d) a look of fear in the eyes upon food presentation. Based on these behaviors the following questions were asked:

1. Is neurological damage the only contributor to oral motor problems in this population?
2. Are there other physical or mechanical reasons for the swallowing difficulties observed in the infant who is NG fed or who also has a tracheostomy?
3. Is there a behavioral component to the swallowing disorder in these infants?

REVIEW OF LITERATURE

Causes of Swallowing Disorders in Infants

The complex coordinated act of swallowing is highly developed in the normal infant and is determined by both autonomic and central nervous system control.[8] Illingworth proposed three main causes of swallowing disorders: (a) gross congenital anatomical defects, e.g., cleft palate, pharyngeal or laryngeal cyst; (b) neuromuscular deficits, e.g., prematurity, cerebral palsy, cranial nerve damage; and (c) acute infective conditions, e.g., esophagitis.[8] DiScipio presented evidence of a fourth cause of dysphagia which he calls conditioned dysphagia.[9] This refers to dysphagia that is acquired and maintained through a behavioral conditioning process and thereby considered a learned disorder. DiScipio proposed that chronic dysphagia may be all or partly related to maladaptive learning, independent of physical causes. He hypothesized that conditioned dysphagia is likely to appear when severe esophageal trauma occurs during the early phases of central nervous system maturation (before five years of age). Trauma to bordering anatomical regions, such as the mouth, chest, and thorax, during concurrent swallowing will also result in conditioned dysphagia. Examples of such traumatic events include intrusive medical procedures, such as NG tube feedings, barium swallow studies, bronchoscopies, and tracheostomies.[9]

The conditioning mechanism as described by DiScipio is illustrated in Figures 1 and 2.[9,10] Physical trauma to the esophagus or bordering areas during intrusive diagnostic or surgical measures is considered the unconditioned aversive stimulus that, when paired temporarily with swallowing, results in conditioned avoidance to swallowing on subsequent, less severe stimulation of the esophagus or mouth (Figure 1). Avoidance responses to swallowing are adaptive behaviors which enable an individual to avoid aversive stimuli or punishment. These behaviors may occur in the presence of proprioceptive and visual stimuli that resemble those present during the trauma. Consequently, oral feeding attempts may act as conditional stimuli resulting in the suppression of swallowing (Figure 2). The introduction of food in the mouth may cause avoidance behaviors, such as gagging, pushing the food away, physical expulsion, or vomiting. When these avoidance behaviors persist long after the probability of presentation of the aversive stimuli is removed, the response is considered a fixed maladaptive habit.

DiScipio recommends deconditioning treatment immediately following the trauma for conditioned dysphagia.[9] Behavior modification methods are used to provide (a) gradual shaping of normal oral feedings using positive reinforcement (small amounts of liquid then pureed foods given initially) and (b) a contingency plan scheduling oral feedings concurrently with tube feedings.

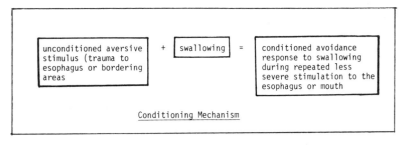

FIGURE 1

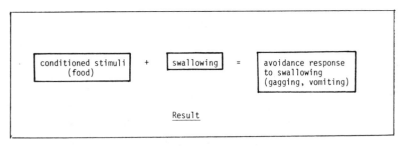

FIGURE 2

Enteral Nutritional Support via Nasogastric and Gastrointestinal Tube Feeding

Greene et al. studied the effects of nocturnal NG tube feedings given at home to fourteen subjects with a variety of chronic diseases.[4] The results indicate nasogastric tube feeding at home to be a safe and economical means of treating and preventing malnutrition in chronic disorders. The purpose of nocturnal NG feedings is to promote oral feeding during the day. Twelve of the fourteen subjects progressed to total oral feedings within a one to three month period.

Van Dyke et al. studied three cases of severe feeding dysfunction in infants with fetal alcohol syndrome.[11] Each subject received total NG tube feedings by four months of age. Intervention consisted of an individualized feeding program aimed at total oral food intake. The feeding program combined oral feeding sessions with the NG or G tube feeding and insured the removal of NG tubes prior to oral feedings. All the subjects displayed difficulty in progressing toward total oral feedings. The authors suggested that irritation caused by the NG tube could have hindered their progress toward oral feedings.

Cataldi-Betcher et al. studied complications occurring in 253 patients treated with enteral nutritional support via tube feedings.[5] There are three categories describing the serious potential complications of tube feedings: (a) gastrointestinal, e.g., nausea, vomiting, diarrhea; (b) mechanical, e.g., aspiration pneumonia from reflux; and (c) metabolic, e.g., serum electrolyte abnormalities, fluid imbalances. Of the 253 patients studied, 30 patients (11.7%) experienced one of the above three complications. Gastrointestinal (GI) complications were most common, followed by mechanical complications. Profuse diarrhea was the most frequent GI complication. Common mechanical complications included lower esophageal sphincter incompetence and reflux of gastric contents, leading to aspiration pneumonia. The use of nasogastric tubes that are too large was also shown to reduce the competency of the esophagogastric sphincter and thus increase the risk of gastric reflux. Furthermore, NG tubes that are too large may cause nasal or esophageal ulceration, pharyngitis, or the formation of a tracheal fistula. Some mechanical complications of G tube feeding include leakage of gastric contents, leading to skin erosion, wound infection, hemorrhage, and tube dislodgement. In this study, Cataldi-

Betcher et al. indicate that although enteral tube feedings are both economical and safe for most patients, health professionals associated with the tube fed patient must be aware of potential tube feeding complications and their management.[5]

Dobie suggested that using small silastic feeding tubes may minimize the risks of reflux esophagitis and nasal and pharyngeal irritation.[12] He also indicated that NG tube feedings are best used as a temporary measure and that indwelling tubes are less irrittating than those taken in and out throughout the day for feedings.

Other complications from enteral tube feedings were indicated by Simon and Handler.[7] They reported that infants who receive NG and G tube feedings for long periods of time may develop oral hypersensitivity from the lack of oral experiences. Behavioral problems may occur during oral feeding attempts as a result of the oral hypersensitivity. Forced feedings by professional staff or family may reinforce the negative attitude toward oral feedings. Intervention for the tube fed infant included initating oral experiences early and encouraging feeding sessions to be relaxed and enjoyable.

Tracheostomies

Wetmore et al. reported pediatric tracheostomy to be a surgical procedure with significant morbidity and mortality.[13] Complications of tracheostomy appear greater in children than adults, especially in cases involving long-term tracheostomy. In a retrospective study of 420 children with pediatric tracheostomy Wetmore et al. identified 49% as having complications.[13] The most frequent early complication was accidental decannulation, followed by pneumonia; the most frequent late complication (after one year) was tracheocutaneous fistula.

Swallowing difficulties in children with tracheostomies were also recognized as significant long-term problems.[13,14] Bonanno reported that on occasion swallowing difficulties were alleviated in some patients upon removal of the tracheostomy tube.[14]

Three possible physiological causes of dysphagia following tracheostomy have been identified.

1. Fixation of the larynx by the tracheostomy tube may occur as a result of the tracheostomy tube anchoring the trachea to the anterior muscles and skin of the neck, causing diminished

laryngeal excursion.[14] During normal swallowing slight elevation and forward movement of the larynx is the most important factor in preventing aspiration.[12] Without laryngeal excursion liquid or food will spill into the larynx and cause tracheal aspiration.

2. The esophagus can be compressed by the tracheal tube.
3. The larynx can become desensitized after the diversion of normal air current through the tracheostomy.[15]

Oral Feeding Intervention

There is relatively little specific information discussed in the literature regarding oral feeding intervention for infants who are tube fed and those with tracheostomies. General guidelines for intervention, proposed by several authors, include the following:

1. Pair oral feeding experiences with the NG or G tube feeding.[9]
2. Begin oral feeding experiences as early as possible when tube feedings have been initiated.[7]
3. Encourage relaxed and enjoyable oral feeding sessions and prevent forced feeding.[7]
4. Grade oral feeding experiences from small amounts to larger amounts.[9]

In summary, the literature indicates there may be both behavioral and physiologic reasons for swallowing and oral feeding difficulties in tube fed infants and those with tracheostomies. Motor incoordination as a result of neurological damage may not be the only reason for oral feeding problems in this population. There is relatively little information in the literature, however, regarding oral feeding intervention for the non-oral feeder.

DISCUSSION

All the possible causes of oral motor problems leading to non-oral feedings must be considered when planning feeding intervention programs for infants who are tube fed and for those with tracheostomies. Evaluation by the occupational therapists should be comprehensive, taking into account both physical and behavioral causes of oral feeding dysfunction.

Physical Causes of Dysfunction

Possible physical factors should be considered when attempting to determine the cause(s) of oral motor dysfunction leading to non-oral feedings.

Neurological Deficits

Some of the most frequent underlying problems causing swallowing and feeding difficulties in infants are neurologic.[16] Some of the problems neurological damage may cause include velopharyngeal incompetence with nasal regurgitation, pharyngeal incoordination, and/or laryngeal incompetence with aspiration.[17]

Clinically, the occupational therapist can readily evaluate the oral preparatory and oral phase of swallowing during a feeding assessment.[6] Observations of how foods or liquids are taken into the mouth and prepared for swallowing can be made. Accurate evaluation of the pharyngeal phase of swallowing by clinical observation is difficult, however. Radiographic procedures, such as modified barium swallow examination, are necessary for examining all the stages of swallowing, including the pharyngeal and esophageal phases. These studies are recommended for infants with swallowing problems and questionable aspiration. If the radiographic examination reveals a significant amount of aspiration, oral feeding attempts may be contraindicated and non-oral feedings may be permanent.[6] The occupational therapists' goal in this case may be limited to oral motor intervention to prevent hypersensitivity and to provide adequate oral hygiene. Depending on the type of swallowing problem, if a minimal amount of aspiration is present, certain dietary measures and positions may help in decreasing aspiration, such as the use of thick foods.

Nasal and/or Pharyngeal Irritation

It is important for the occupational therapist to be aware that nasal and/or pharyngeal irritation may develop as a result of NG tube feedings. Thus, the presence of the NG tube may cause discomfort during swallowing and as a result inhibit oral feedings. There are three main approaches used in NG tube feedings: (a) inserting and withdrawing the NG tube for each feeding, (b) an indwelling NG tube (left in all day), and (c) nocturnal NG feedings. Inserting and withdrawing the NG tube for every feeding may be harmful because this provides frequent noxious stimuli to the oral region and may promote nasal and/or pharyngeal irritation and conditioned dysphagia. Removal of the NG tube during oral feeding experiences however, may be beneficial in promoting swallowing and pleasurable experiences during these times. The use of indwelling NG tubes may be a preferred method for NG tube feedings to minimize noxious experiences around the oral region, pharyngeal irritation, and conditioned dysphagia.[12] Nocturnal feedings may be helpful in preventing the noxious stimuli of the tube during the day, allowing positive oral feeding experiences.

Tracheostomy Complications

Occupational therapists should be aware of the possible physical complications that may occur with tracheostomy placement, which may cause significant swallowing problems and subsequent aspiration. For example laryngeal excursion may be limited from the tracheal tube and cause aspiration upon swallowing. This information would be critical when planning intervention. Radiographic measures, along with close communication with the physician, can assist in identifying these possible complications.

Oral Hypersensitivity

Hypersensitivity to touch around and in the mouth may result from disuse of the oral mechanism for feeding. Infants who are given enteral nutritional support via NG or G tubes often lack adequate oral tactile input to the mouth. Without early and continued oral motor intervention, even when oral feedings are contraindicated, the tube fed infant may develop this hypersensitivity. Touch to these areas may be perceived as noxious stimuli.

Behavioral Causes of Dysfunction

Conditioned Dysphagia

Conditioned dysphagia may occur from the trauma related to NG feedings or tracheostomy placement. This purposeful avoidance of swallowing may be present without actual physical dysfunction of the swallowing mechanism. If the results of swallowing studies rule out dysfunction of the swallowing mechanism and the infant has a history of trauma occurring around the oral region, conditioned dysphagia may be the likely cause of swallowing problems. Symptoms of this condition were described in the literature review.

Once conditioned dysphagia is identified, the occupational therapist must consider whether the unconditioned aversive stimuli can be removed. Since the NG tube can serve as an unconditioned aversive stimulus, frequent placement and removal should be avoided. Also, if tube feedings are predicted to last more than one to three months, the G tube may be indicated as the best means of enteral nutritional support. Once the aversive stimuli of NG tube feedings is removed, perhaps attempts toward oral feedings will be more successful.

Unconditioned aversive stimuli leading to conditioned dysphagia may also occur as a result of tracheostomy placement. Suctioning of the tracheal tube may be aversive for some infants and should be avoided prior to and during feeding. Any of the possible physical complications of tracheostomy, such as pressure of the tracheal tube against the esophagus, may cause discomfort during swallowing and subsequently lead to conditioned dysphagia. If the complication can not be alleviated by medical intervention, the goal of total oral feeding is most likely not a realistic or appropriate one until the tracheostomy tube is removed.

Touch around and/or in the mouth during feeding may be considered aversive stimuli for those infants who are hypersensitive to this type of touch. A forceful approach to feeding in this case may cause conditioned dysphagia. The aversive stimuli, touch, should not be completely removed. However, a graded approach in providing oral input is indicated.

If the aversive stimuli can not be removed for a period of time, it is important for the occupational therapist to provide as many pleasurable oral experiences as possible for the infant, so that there may be some balance of positive and negative experiences. Once the aversive stimuli are removed or decreased as much as possible, an oral motor and feeding intervention program should be provided early, gradually, and in a consistent manner. If the child is cared for at home, it is extremely important that the parents follow up consistently with the feeding program (at least three sessions per day).

Social Environment

Often parents of infants receiving non-oral feedings are strongly committed toward helping their child progress to total oral feedings. According to Morris, oral feeding sessions may develop into high stress times for both the feeder and the infant resulting in (a) limited bonding and (b) a breakdown in communication between the feeder and infant.[18] These problems often happen because mechanical issues are stressed instead of communication and social issues.[18]

SUGGESTED TREATMENT STRATEGIES

Early Referral and Intervention

Intervention for infants with oral motor problems and for those who have had invasive medical procedures around the oral area should be initiated as soon as possible. For this to occur it is important that there be close communication between the medical staff and occupational therapist regarding the treatment needs of this special population. Often times referrals for oral motor and feeding intervention are delayed until the medical staff feels oral feedings can be initiated. During this period the infant may have received few, if any, positive oral experiences, resulting in the development of hypersensitivity. At the time of referral for oral motor and feeding intervention the parents and therapist may suddenly feel pressured from the medical staff to help the child quickly progress to total oral feedings.[18] The stress of this situation may cause increased resistive behavior by the child. The end result of this situation may be feelings of failure by all the parties involved.

This situation is avoidable. Education of the medical staff regarding the services occupational therapists can offer for non-oral feeders must be provided on an ongoing basis to (a) obtain early referrals and (b) clarify misperceptions regarding oral feeding intervention. Progression from non-oral to total oral feedings is usually a slow one. Physicians, nurses, parents, and therapists must be aware of this and thus lower their initial expectations. Initially, treatment expectations should emphasize *qualitative* aspects of oral motor and feeding versus *quantity* of food taken in, especially since the infant is receiving adequate enteral nutritional support via the NG or G tube.[18] The therapist and parent should strive to make the feeding sessions relaxed and enjoyable with improved positive communication and sensorimotor experiences for the infant.

Enhance Normal Posture and Movement

Abnormal muscle tone and movement patterns may be present in the infant with neurological damage. Hyperextension of the head is an example of an abnormal movement pattern this usually leads to oral motor problems, such as tongue retraction, lip retraction, and jaw thrust. The occupational therapist must be aware of how total body patterns influence the mouth. Handling and positioning should enhance normal posture and movement, along with midline control of the head, neck, and trunk.

Decrease Oral Hypersensitivity and Conditioned Dysphagia

Morris suggests playful stimulation around the face and mouth instead of mechanical desensitization programs for the infant who is (a) fearful of touch around the oral region and/or (b) hypersensitive to the tactile input.[18] Touching and caressing can be provided with the therapist's or child's hands or with interesting toys having a variety of textures. Songs and games can accompany the graded touch to encourage its enjoyment. The infant will most often accept oral tactile input that is self initiated prior to accepting it from another. It is important for the therapist and parents to let the child guide how much oral tactile input is tolerable. The child's nonverbal cues can easily indicate likes and dislikes, such as smiles, frowns, increased tone, crying, and pursed lips.[18] Careful observation of these nonverbal cues signals alteration of the treatment approach. Graded oral stimulation should occur frequently and consistently throughout the day, both during and after oral feeding sessions.

Facilitate a Rhythmical Suck and Swallow

According to Morris the suck or suckle will facilitate a swallow response.[18] Therefore, in treatment to improve swallowing it may be helpful to increase sucking.

Many infants stop sucking from the bottle once NG tube feedings are initiated. The presence of the NG tube may cause discomfort during suck-swallow. Attempts to facilitate sucking from the bottle may be unsuccessful due to (a) conditioned dysphagia; (b) hypersensitivity of the tongue to touch; and (c) poor tongue configuration, tone, and movement. All three of these problems may need to be addressed before sucking from the bottle is an accepted and successful experience. If these problems are present, persistent attempts at bottle feeding may in fact develop into an invasive experience for the infant and a failure experience for the feeder. The goal of sucking from a bottle may be premature at this time.

There are various ways the therapist can facilitate sucking without using a bottle, however. The use of the therapist's or infant's fingers or soft, pliable toys around and in the mouth during play may help prepare the infant for touch in the mouth. Once the infant is accepting touch in the mouth, the therapist can then help to improve tongue configuration, tone, and movement. Infants with abnormal tone often have tongues that are hypotonic, thick, or bunched, which is different from the normal tongue that has a flattened, cupped configuration.[18] To normalize tone and configuration of the tongue, Morris suggests downward patting on the tongue with the index finger. Stroking the lateral borders of the tongue may facilitate lateral tongue movements.[18] Sucking may then be facilitated by providing a rhythmical stroking of the tongue with a down and forward pressure of the index finger.[18] The advantage of the therapist using his/her finger is that changes in the infant's tongue can more readily be felt than if a toy or nipple is used. Small tastes of juices or pureed foods can also be used during these activities. Once the infant begins sucking on the therapist's finger, sucking from the bottle may be a possibility. However, if the bottle is persistently rejected by the infant, the cup may be the most appropriate alternative.

Gradually Progress From Non-Oral to Oral Feedings

A gradual progression from non-oral to oral feedings is important so that oral feeding sessions do not become invasive and negative experiences for the infant. The use of utensils (bottles, spoons, and cups) should be introduced gradually and only when the infant responds positively to them. If utensils are rejected, small amounts of food may be introduced by finger. Also, it may be helpful to encourage the infant to initiate hand to mouth patterns while touching and playing with food. Self-initiated feeding experiences may be the least threatening for the infant. A graded introduction of food may begin with drops of water, then flavored water given by finger, next dabs of pureed food, followed by thickened pureed foods, then mashed table foods.[18] Solid finger foods should be introduced early (7–8 months) to encourage biting and chewing behaviors. The infant should be watched closely during these times to prevent choking, if a large piece breaks off. As the child begins to accept foods, it is important to introduce a variety of feeding experiences with liquids, mashed soft foods, and solid chewing foods. Throughout the oral feeding intervention program the therapist must emphasize *quality* feeding experiences as well as increased *quantity* of food taken in. The infant not only must develop a good suck-swallow but also adequate lip, cheek, tongue, and jaw control for biting and chewing a variety of foods.

Monitor Tube Feedings

Clinically it has been noted that the amount of food received by tube has a significant effect on the success of oral feeding sessions. If the infant is receiving more than adequate amounts of food by tube, oral feedings may be rejected. It is important for there to be adequate time intervals between feedings to allow the child to experience a feeling of hunger and then a feeling of fullness after an oral feeding. Planning the amount and schedule of food intake should be closely coordinated with the dietician, parent, and physician.

CASE EXAMPLE

The following case example describes an occupational therapy intervention program for a tube fed infant and the progression from non-oral to oral feedings.

Brian is an 11 month old boy who was born with a congenital heart defect (Tetrology of Fallot). He has mild low tone and minimal developmental delay. After several cyanotic attacks as an infant, Brian was hospitalized at 2 months of age and underwent open heart surgery. During this time NG tube feedings were initiated and bottle feedings ceased. Occupational therapy for oral motor and feeding intervention was initiated 3 months later, around the time of hospital discharge. Since then, Brian received approximately 6 months of home-based occupational therapy with one hour sessions, twice per week. Primary treatment emphasis has been in the area of oral motor and feeding development.

At the time of initial evaluation, Brian received total nutritional support via an NG tube that was left in place. He demonstrated symptoms of conditioned dysphagia by physically refusing food, gagging, and vomiting. He also indicated oral hypersensitivity by showing displeasure with touch around and in the mouth and by gagging with touch to the anterior and middle of the tongue. His tongue was thick and bunched and he was unable to suck.

Treatment emphasized (a) positive and graded oral tactile experiences with the therapist's and child's hands or soft toys; (b) facilitation of normal tongue configuration, tone, and movement; (c) introduction of drops of liquid or small dabs of pureed food by finger to the front of the mouth; (d) handling to facilitate mid-range head control; and (e) close communication with the parents to ensure consistent follow up at home. After 3 months of intervention the *quality* of oral motor experiences improved. Brian began to enjoy touch around and in his mouth and to actively explore toys with his mouth. His tongue appeared less thick and bunched and more mobile. Progress towards increasing the *quantity* of food taken orally was minimal, however. Brian swallowed approximately one tablespoon of pureed foods given by finger in a 30-minute session. He frequently vomited after the feeding session.

Although Brian made some improvements during the time he was fed by the NG tube, there seemed to be several complications resulting from its placement. First, this was an invasive procedure, possibly causing conditioned dysphagia. Brian gagged and cried when he observed the NG tube approach his face for placement. Reflux appeared to be another complication; he vomited regularly throughout the day. The presence of the NG tube also seemed to prevent suck-swallow. Lastly, it was felt that he developed nasopharyngeal irritation due to the long duration of NG tube placement. Due to these complications and limited progress in *quantity* of food intake, it appeared that the NG tube was hindering the progression to total oral feeding. Brian had developed an interest in mouthing toys and teething biscuits and accepted small amounts of pureed foods, but resistance to swallowing continued to be a problem. After a team meeting with the physician, parent, and occupational therapist it was decided that gastrostomy tube placement was indicated. This would allow the aversive stimulus of the NG tube to be removed.

Brian was hospitalized for 4 days to have the gastrostomy procedure. During those 4 days he received intravenous feedings.

By the 5th day, upon release from the hospital, he demonstrated obvious behaviors indicating hunger, excessive mouthing of toys and objects. Within three days he was eating 1.5 ounces of baby food by spoon in 10–15 minute sessions, three times per day. He swallowed foods fluidly and with ease. Brian also drank small amounts of liquids by cup and continued to teeth on firm cookies. All vomiting and gagging completely stopped.

During Brian's first week with the G tube feedings the amounts given by tube were gradually increased to approximately 15 ounces more per day than what he was given by NG tube, to increase his weight gain. After one week of G tube feedings *all* oral feeding intake ceased. Brian began to demonstrate significant avoidance behaviors during oral feeding sessions, including (a) crying, (b) pushing food away, (c) maintained tongue retraction and mouth opening to prevent swallowing, and (d) falling asleep during the feeding session. Brian also began to vomit several times per day. This change in oral feeding behavior was perplexing. It seemed the only variable that could have influenced this change was the increase in G tube feedings. After the occupational therapist consulted with the physician and dietitian, the G tube feedings were decreased approximately 10–15 ounces per day. Again, after 3–4 days he began to accept oral feedings and stopped vomiting throughout the day. Within one month the oral feedings increased to 4 ounces, three times per day, with G tube feedings given at night.

Brian continues to receive occupational therapy to improve quality and quantity of oral feeding with the ultimate goal of total oral feedings.

SUMMARY

The literature indicates that neurological damage may not be the only cause of oral motor and swallowing problems in the tube fed infant and the infant with tracheostomy. Certain behavioral and/or physical complications of nasogastric feedings and pediatric tracheostomy may also cause swallowing and oral feeding problems. Occupational therapists working with infants of this special population must be aware of these possible complications and adapt intervention accordingly. Treatment strategies were discussed and then illustrated by a case example.

REFERENCES

1. Clark PN, Allen AS: Occupational Therapy for Children. St. Louis: The C.V. Mosby Company, 1985, p 224

2. Scherzer AL, Tscharnuter IT: Early Diagnosis and Therapy in Cerebral Palsy: A Primer on Infant Developmental Problems. New York: Marcel Dekker, Inc., 1982, p 57

3. Logan WJ, Bosma JF: Oral and pharyngial dysphagia in infancy. *Pediatr Clin N Am* 14: 47–61, 1967

4. Greene HL, Helinek GL, Folk CC, Courtney M, Thompson S, MacDonell RC, Lukens JN: Nasogastric tube feeding at home: A method for adjunctive nutritional support of malnourished patients. *Am J Clin Nutr* 34: 1131–1138, 1981

5. Cataldi-Betcher EL, Seltzer MH, Slocum BA, Jones KW: Complications occurring during enteral nutrition support: A prospective study. *JPEN* 7: 546–552, 1983

6. Logemann J: Evaluation and Treatment of Swallowing Disorders. San Diego: College-Hill Press, Inc., 1983, p 236, 28–31

7. Simon B, Handler SD: The speech pathologist and management of children with tracheostomies. *J Otolaryngol* 10: 440–448, 1981

8. Illingworth RS: Sucking and swallowing difficulties in infancy: Diagnostic problem of dysphagia. *Dis Childh* 44: 644–655, 1969

9. DiScipio WJ, Kaslon K, Ruben RJ: Traumatically acquired conditioned dysphagia in children. *Ann Otolaryngol* 87: 509–514, 1978

10. DiScipio WJ, Kaslon K: Conditioned dysphagia in cleft palate children after pharyngeal flap surgery. *Psychom Med* 44: 247–257, 1982

11. VanDyke DC, Mackay L, Ziaylek EN: Management of severe feeding dysfunction in children with fetal alcohol syndrome. *Clin Pediatr* 21: 336–339, 1982

12. Dobie RA: Rehabilitation of swallowing disorders. *AFP* 17: 84–95, 1978

13. Wetmore RF, Handler SD, Potsic WP: Pediatric tracheostomy: Experiences during the past decade. *Ann Otol Rhinol Laryngol* 91: 628–632, 1982

14. Bonanno PC: Swallowing dysfunction after tracheostomy. *Ann Surg* 174: 29–33, 1971

15. Feldman SA, Deal CW, Urquhart W: Disturbance of swallowing after tracheostomy. *Lancet* 1: 954–955, 1966

16. Fisher SE, Painter M, Milmore G: Swallowing disorders in infancy. *Ped Clin N Am* 28: 845–853, 1981

17. Williams DJ, Mitchell DP: Pharynogoesophageal dysphagia in infancy. *Int J Pediatr Otorhinolaryngol* 2: 231–242, 1980

18. Morris SE: Unpublished workshop notes: The normal acquisition of oral feeding skills: Implications for assessment and treatment. Orlando, Florida, 1983

Behavioral Feeding Disorders in Young Children: An Occupational Therapy Frame of Reference

Rick Denton, MA, OTR

ABSTRACT. Young children with behavioral feeding disorders are commonly seen in occupational therapy practice. This paper, based on clinical experience with these children, presents an expanded frame of reference which may be utilized in treatment. The combined use of food as play and treatment of choice is addressed and viewed from learning, developmental, psychodynamic and humanistic perspectives. Possible etiologies of these specific feeding behaviors are discussed.

Occupational therapists are accustomed to evaluating and treating children with feeding deficits of a physical or neuromotor nature. Feeding problems which are behaviorally oriented however, present the occupational therapist with a different kind of challenge. Occupational therapists may need further understanding regarding the incidence of maladaptive feeding behaviors and the availability of treatment approaches which have potential to address these problems. Maladaptive feeding behaviors are those which are poorly suited for normal physical and emotional growth to occur. They may include volitionally controlled absence of self feeding, aversive reactions to the touch or sight of food, or highly unusual food preferences such as intake of one type of food to the exclusion of all others. Frequently the occupational therapist is called in on such cases to evaluate feeding difficulties which appear to the

Rick Denton is Assistant Professor of Occupational Therapy, Louisiana State University Medical Center, New Orleans, LA.

This article appears jointly in *Occupational Therapy for People With Eating Dysfunctions* (The Haworth Press, Inc., 1986) and Occupational Therapy in Health Care, Volume 3, Number 2 (Summer 1986).

81

referral source to be related to oral motor dysfunction. Since evaluation is essential to treatment planning, a thorough oral motor assessment as well as feeding history are completed and are usually complimentary to a standard developmental evaluation. An assessment protocol such as one described earlier by Denton[1] may be especially useful with this population. Occupational therapists need to be prepared to deal with evaluation results which indicate normal oral motor functions but atypical feeding behaviors. Lewis, an occupational therapist, highlights the need for such preparation, as 40% of parents responding to her questionnaire regarding feeding techniques and management, identified "behavior problems" as an area of concern.[2]

ETIOLOGIES OF BEHAVIORAL FEEDING DISORDERS

Although occupational therapists have recently begun to address behavioral problems relating to feeding,[3] relatively few sources identify the possible etiologies of these disorders. O'Neil and colleagues,[4,5] non-occupational therapists, have attempted to specifically address behavior management techniques for these feeding disorders, but do not fully identify etiologies. Morris and Tscharnuter[6,7] present some valuable information about interpersonal aspects of feeding but focus primarily on physically impaired infants and their caretakers, and the complicating effects upon the feeding process. There is very little information available in the child psychiatry literature which specifically addresses psychosocial feeding disorders. These behaviors are lumped into nebulous categories such as "Atypical Eating Disorders"[8] or Habit Disorders,[9] also known as "Transient Situational Disturbances of Childhood". Freedman et al.[10] in their discussion of related behavior disorders of childhood, state that "the diversity of these conditions" prevents specific etiological hypotheses to be made and that causation needs to be investigated on an individual case basis.

Occupational therapists have potential to provide helpful intervention guidelines, by attempting to identify possible causative factors or existing conditions which foster the development or prolongation of behavior feeding disorders.

The effects of neuromotor and sensory deficits upon the feeding process appear readily understood, yet many toddlers and preschoolers who are referred to occupational therapy for oral motor assessment, and who present with behavior feeding disorders, are frequently those children who are described as having had "feeding difficulties since birth". As infants these children typically were premature, had congential malformations such as cleft palate, presented with cardiac conditions or were identified as having suffered perinatal trauma. Many also lacked adquate oral input due to alternate feeding methods such as gastrostomies, NG tubes or hyperalimentation. Parents often provide information during the feeding history which indicates they were never instructed in feeding facilitation or that they were provided with questionable intervention strategies such as cutting holes in nipples or using "infafeeders". They also may not have been told of the importance of continued sensory oral input when alternate feeding methods are being used.[11] These practices and others such as force feeding may lead to increased caretaker-child stress surrounding feeding events, the child's negative association with food or eating, decreased growth with possible malnutrition, and in certain cases subsequent "failure to thrive" (F.T.T.).[12] Many young children with maladaptive feeding behaviors are diagnosed F.T.T. due to their insufficient height and weight for age.[1,13] Early identification and appropriate treatment in infancy may greatly reduce the risk of behavioral feeding disorders developing in the preschool years.

Maladaptive feeding behaviors may also be observed in physically normal young children who are experiencing environmental stress or are in situations where food becomes a means of emotional control.[14] These children tend to develop unusual food preferences such as willingness to eat chips, swects or crackers to the exclusion of fruit, meat or vegetables. This too may lead to more coercive parental measures (such as force feeding) to ensure nutrient intake by the child. This may spiral into a non-compromising struggle between the parents and child, resulting in significant negative associations with food and eating and the occurrence of severe maladaptive behaviors such as vomiting, gagging, breath holding or spitting at the sight, touch or taste of food. Feeding behaviors such as these are also effective attention seeking maneuvers!

Whether maladaptive feeding behaviors are a result of unidentified or inadequately treated infant feeding problems, control issues between caretaker(s) and child, or are attention seeking devices, their remediation is tantamount to enhancing physical and emotional growth.

FRAME OF REFERENCE

Mosey[15] states that a frame of reference is a linking structure between theory and practice and should be one that is readily useable. The structure for the frame of reference suggested here, is based on her model, but organized specifically to address behavioral feeding problems (see Tables 1 and 2).

TREATMENT RATIONALE

The severe nature of behavioral feeding disorders often creates increased familial distress and may ultimately predispose the child to physical abuse.[16,17] These children are often hospitalized after prolonged feeding difficulties and substantial growth failure. The occupational therapist, skilled in assessing behavioral as well as the neuromotor components of feeding, may be a valuable team member in the identification and treatment of these children.

The occupational therapy frame of reference suggested here utilizes play as treatment viewed from learning, developmental, psychodynamic and humanistic perspectives. Because play is a primary occupation of the child it appears to be the nucleus to actively resolving maladaptive feeding behaviors. Children generally respond to play but they may not have sufficient cognitive skills to participate in verbal treatment methods.

Eysenck sees symptoms as being evidence of faulty learning.[18] Vomiting, gagging or breath holding at the sight of food would in this case be symptoms. Such a child has learned to associate foods with displeasure. The extinction of these behaviors is achieved by pairing foods and eating with pleasure. Play is used as both the treatment and as the reward for successful approximations at touching, tasting or actual eating of foods. If a child is hesitantly finger painting with pudding and attempts to clean his/her soiled fingers by licking them, he/she may be given an immediate chance to participate in a play activity (such as riding in the net swing, or playing in water) which has been previously determined to be highly rewarding.

Developmentally, sensory-motor play is viewed by Piaget as movements in space, handling objects and practicing control via exploration and manipulation.[19] Piaget stresses the importance of this type of play including its oral, tactile and kinesthetic properties

Table 1
Continuums and Behaviors Indicative of Dysfunction

1. Feeding Issues:
   a. absent self feeding (volitional absence or due to ng tube, gastrostomy, force feeding, etc.)
   b. aversive reactions to sight of food (crying, head turning, refusal, pushing away)
   c. avoidance of touching food (clean eaters whose caretakers are often "antimessy")
   d. negative associations with food and eating (learned behavior)
   e. decreased contact with foods of varying tastes and textures (may dislike oral tactile input, may be hypersensitive orally, may develop unusual food preferences)

2. Psychosocial Issues:
   a. deficient sensory motor play behaviors (may be related to environmental limitations or may exhibit delayed play skills especially those which require manual control or involve tactile processing)
   b. lack of active choice making (due to force feeding or infafeeder use)
   c. frequent display of maladaptive behavior(s) (gagging, vomiting, squirreling, breath holding, etc.)
   d. decreased basic need fulfillment (lack of nourishment)
   e. inability to appropriately master environmental demands (seeks attention, gains control via effective, yet inappropriate means)

3. Physical Growth Issues:
   a. inadequate caloric intake
   b. height and weight below age expectancy

as components of early relationship development. Children with behavioral feeding disorders who often avoid touching and tasting foods to the point of becoming malnourished may need to be reintroduced to sensory-motor play and especially to activities which utilize food and cooking themes that may be rich in sensory variation, manipulation and exploration. Suggested activities might

Table 2
Postulates Regarding Change

1. Feeding Issues may be resolved by:

    a. pairing foods with pleasurable activity
    b. play activities which use food items as the medium of play rather
       than sustenance
    c. play activities which encourage varied oral and tactile sensory
       experiences
    d. activities which encourage the gross and fine motor patterns
       characteristic of self feeding

2. Psychosocial Issues may be addressed via:

    a. separation of child and caretaker during meal time or feeding
       activity
    b. decreased emphasis on food consumption
    c. sensory motor play experiences which involve food or cooking themes
    d. opportunities to make choices, be in control
    e. provision of positive reinforcement for successful attempts at, or
       actual oral intake

*3. Physical Growth Issues may be resolved via:

    a. elimination of maladaptive feeding behaviors and the establishment
       of self directed feeding
    b. generalized feeding behaviors resulting in adequate caloric intake
       and growth

*This is a general postulate which is directly dependent upon feeding and
psychosocial issues resolution

include stacking cubes of cheese, mixing yogurt in a play blender, or engaging in a game of "cherry tomato hockey", using carrot sticks to push the fake puck across the table. This is another means by which foods and eating can be positively paired, incorporating important sensory motor characteristics necessary for the establishment of self feeding.

Freudian theory states that play enables the child to master disturbing events by active participation rather than being a passive or helpless spectator.[20] Using play in this manner appears useful with the child who has been force fed or who has lacked opportunities to appropriately master environmental demands. Examples of activities using this framework might be encouraging the child to mix, mash, pour, tear and shake food/liquid items of their own creation, and allowing them to pretend feed stuffed animals or dolls or feeding occasional spoonfuls or bites of food to the therapist.

Humanistic thought espouses self actualization or the fulfilling of ones highest potential.[21] Maslow states that self actualization cannot take place without basic need fulfillment (defined as adequate food and water). As the child is provided sensory-motor play experiences, opportunities to master environmental demands and learns to associate foods with pleasure, the child becomes self directed in the fulfilling of basic needs and thus closer to self actualization. It is not until this level of learning has been achieved that physical growth can occur without the need for immediate reinforcement.

TREATMENT IMPLEMENTATION

Treatment utilizing the theoretical principles previously discussed should be flexible enough to allow for individuality. One child may progress quite rapidly while another may need extra time to work through the sensory aspects of foods during play. Initially with the hospitalized child therapy sessions are typically held at meal times without the parents in attendance. Faulty learning includes having negatively associated parents with the stress that mealtimes usually produce. Parents frequently need to be involved in counseling or training services provided by other professionals to deal with their own frustration, anger and guilt, and sometimes to improve their parenting skills in general. They are introduced to the occupational therapy regime when the child has begun to self feed and when they have been taught by the therapist suggested strategies for replicating the treatment program. Nursing and dietary staff support are essential in carrying out modified feeding plans in the therapist's absence.

Children appear to respond better to this treatment approach if they are hungry. This means that children with unusual food preferences should not be allowed to consume non-nutritious snacks in between scheduled therapy sessions and it is recommended that children who are usually fed by ancillary means, such as gastrostomies, have their feedings scheduled after treatment sessions.

Treatment is advocated being held at least daily and in three phases. *Phase one* treatment is oriented towards associating foods with pleasurable experience. Children are not required to eat nor are foods presented as actual edible items. Activities may include floating carrot sailboats in water, playing with pretend foods such as erasers which replicate fruits in shape, color and smell, or playing Mr. Potato Head with an apple instead of a plastic pretend potato. The therapists imagination is the only limit in creating activities which allow food to be used playfully rather than as sustenance.

In *phase two*, therapy activities enable the child to deal with both sensory aspects of food as well as fostering appropriate opportunities for control and manipulation. Suggested activities may include stringing natural wheat circles or pretzels onto cooked pasta strands, pushing bananas or mashed potatoes through a Playdough factory or making designs from thickened yogurt or pudding that is scooped into, then squeezed out of a cake decorating tool. It is in this phase also where the child is encouraged to feed the therapist or stuffed animals and approximations of self feeding are usually observed. Reinforcement for such attempts should be individualized based on evaluation results.[1] To one child a ride on a scooter down the ramp may be highly reinforcing, to another blowing bubbles, hitting a balloon or playing dress-up may be motivating.

The emphasis of treatment in *phase three* is aimed at increasing oral input via play with whistles, bubble pipes, party blowers and musical toys. Deep oral pressure activities are also used via puppet and roughhouse play with the therapist. The child in this phase is also encouraged to partake in playful contests such as receiving a reward for winning a chewing/swallowing game, with the therapist as competitor. The child at this phase has characteristically begun to self feed with much fewer reinforcers needed.

As the child progresses through the treatment program generalized feeding behaviors are hopefully established, while parents are educated regarding new methods of interaction at feeding time, normal sensory aspects of feeding and ways to reinforce appropriate behavior(s). This treatment approach has proved to be clinically useful, often resulting in physical growth for the child as well as facilitating increased understanding and management of feeding activities by the parents.

SUMMARY

This paper devises a frame of reference occupational therapists may utilize with children who have behavioral feeding disorders. The etiologies, behaviors and activities addressed are derived from clinical occupational therapy practice. The frame of reference is intended to guide pertinent yet previously unorganized information, into a useable intervention tool.

REFERENCES

1. Denton R: An occupational therapy assessment protocol for infants and toddlers who fail to thrive. *AJOT*, in print

2. Lewis JA: Effectiveness of parents training for feeding intervention: The parents' perspective. *AOTA Developmental Disabilities Special Interest Section Newsletter* 7:1–2, 1984

3. Coley IL, Procter SA: Behavioral problems in eating and self feeding. In, Occupational Therapy for Children. P Clark and A Allen. St. Louis: C.V. Mosby Co., 234–236, 1985

4. O'Neil SM: Management of mealtime behaviors. In, Nutrition in Infancy and Childhood, P Pipes. St. Louis: C.V. Mosby Co., 372–381, 1985

5. O'Neil SM, et al.: Behavioral Approaches to Children with Developmental Delays. St. Louis: The C.V. Mosby Co., 1977

6. Morris SE: Interpersonal aspects of feeding problems. In, Oral Motor Function and Dysfunction in Children, J. Wilson, Editor. Chapel Hill, N.C.: Univ. of N.C., Dept. of P.T.

7. Scherzer A, Tscharnuter I: Early Diagnosis and Therapy in Cerebral Palsy. New York: Marcel Dekker Inc., 1982

8. Diagnostic and Statistical Manual of Mental Disorders. Washington D.C.: American Psychiatric Association, 1980

9. Psychopathological Disorders in Childhood: Theoretical Considerations and a Proposed Classification. New York: Group for the Advancement of Psychiatry, 1966

10. Freedman AM, et al.: Modern Synopsis of Comprehensive Textbook of Psychiatry. Baltimore: Williams and Wilkins Company, 1051–1054, 1976

11. Beratis S, Kolb R: Development of a child with long lasting deprivation of oral feeding. *J of Am Acad of Child Psych* 20:53–64, 1981

12. Casey PH: Failure to thrive: A reconceptualization. *J Dev and Beh Ped* 4:63–66, 1983

13. Powell GF, Low J: Behavior in nonorganic failure to thrive. *J of Dev Beh Ped* 4:26–33, 1983

14. Howard B: Nutritional support of the developmentally disabled child. In, Textbook of Pediatric Nutrition. Suskind R, New York: Raven Press, 1981

15. Mosey AC: Exploration of frames of reference. In, Occupational Therapy Configuration of a Profession. New York: Raven Press, 1981

16. Gaensbauer JJ, Sands K: Distorted affective communications in abused/neglected infants and their potential impact on caretakers. *J Am Acad Child Psych* 2:236–250, 1979

17. Milowe ID, Lourie RS: The child's role in the battered child syndrome. *J Ped* 65:1079–1081, 1984

18. Eysenck HJ: Abnormal Psychology, Reading in Theory and Research. Belmont CA: Brooks Cole Publishing, 1981

19. Fong BC, Resnick MR: The Child, Development Through Adolescence. Menlo Park CA: Benjamin/Cummings Publishing, 1980

20. Schaefer C: (Editor) The Therapeutic Use of Child's Play. New York: Jason Aronson Inc., 1976

21. Millar S: The Psychology of Play. Middlesex England: Penguin Books, 1971

The Role of the Itinerant Occupational Therapist in Conducting Feeding Programs for Multi-Handicapped Children in a County School System

Ruth Strauss, OTR

ABSTRACT. Itinerant occupational therapists working in the school system encounter many problems when initiating and conducting feeding programs for their multi-handicapped students. The occupational therapist provides direct treatment or consultative services to best meet the needs of her students and most efficiently and effectively utilize her treatment time. This paper describes feeding training programs and a case history to illustrate some feeding problems encountered by itinerant occupational therapists and how they have been handled.

Eating is a vital function necessary for life. Whether one is being fed or feeds himself, physical, emotional, and social processes are involved. With handicapped children of varied diagnoses and ages, feeding is a critical problem in development frequently encountered by the occupational therapist. As a result of PL 94-142, increased numbers of children are being treated by occupational therapists in the schools. Thus having high caseloads and limited time in

Ruth Strauss is Department Manager, Occupational Therapy-Pediatric Contracts, Easter Seal Society of DeSoto, Manatee and Sarasota Counties, Inc., Happiness House Rehabilitation Center, Sarasota, FL and has practiced pediatric occupational therapy for nine years in hospital and school settings.

The author would like to acknowledge Molly Boardman, OTR, Mary Ellen Brown, OTR, and Diane Palmer, OTR, who were staff therapists in the Occupational Therapy-Pediatric Contracts Department at Easter Seal Society of DeSoto, Manatee and Sarasota Counties, Inc., Happiness House Rehabilitation Center, Sarasota FL at the time this article was written.

This article appears jointly in *Occupational Therapy for People With Eating Dysfunctions* (The Haworth Press, Inc., 1986) and *Occupational Therapy in Health Care*, Volume 3, Number 2 (Summer 1986).

91

schedules to address feeding needs, therapists find that early intervention and remediation have become even more essential to meet the many needs of both physically and mentally handicapped children.

Occupational therapists have long been involved in evaluation and treatment of children with problems of oral-motor coordination and feeding skill deficits. This paper describes feeding programs developed and implemented by occupational therapists at three sites within the Sarasota County, Florida school system. Occupational therapy services are contracted from Easter Seal Society of DeSoto, Manatee and Sarasota Counties, Inc., Happiness House Rehabilitation Center by the School Board's Department of Exceptional Student Education and by Children's Haven and Adult Center. Since each therapist travels to several settings, it is important that they quickly identify the most effective way to meet the daily feeding needs of their students. As part of the interdisciplinary team, this essentially means the occupational therapists must provide both direct services to students and consultation to those regularly on-site with a goal of helping children develop new skills and then carry them over into daily use.

In the descriptions to follow, the general rationales for feeding training programs in each site will be presented indicating both goals and strategies used, how the occupational therapist relates to other staff in carrying them out and some indication of outcomes. This will be followed by one illustrative case history/study along with general recommendations for providing occupational therapy feeding services in multiple settings.

SETTING A

This is a public school for trainable mentally handicapped children ages 9–13 years. The feeding program initiated by the occupational therapist was conducted in the school cafeteria during regular food service times. The occupational therapist was present twice a week during the one-half hour lunch period to work with the teacher and aide in carrying out recommended programs. She did evaluations on each child periodically, set up the program routines and then spent on-site visits in follow-up consultation with other staff and assisting in a one to one situation as needed.

Since most of the children involved already had basic self-feeding skills, the program was directed to improving the quality of those skills, to increase the flow of students in the cafeteria and encourage generally acceptable social behaviors. Specific goals for the group as a whole emphasized social skills. The strengths and weaknesses of each child were considered prior to establishing the following group goals which encouraged learning to:

1. Remain quiet and in place in cafeteria line
2. Hold food tray properly
3. Eat at an appropriate speed
4. Remain seated and facing table during meal
5. Chew with mouth closed
6. Interact with others at table in a socially acceptable manner
7. Empty and return food tray

Adaptive equipment was kept at a minimum with this group. Dycem helped stabilize the cafeteria tray or plate. With some students, it was necessary to remove the food from the partitioned trays on which the cafeteria served food to a plate (regular, scoop dish, or plate with plate guard) for ease and independence in scooping. Built-up handle spoons were used in several cases to assist with grasp. Physical prompting and verbal cuing, forward and backward chaining and behavior modification techniques were other strategies used in this feeding setting. When working with a feeding program, it is obvious that the food itself becomes a primary reinforcement. Social reinforcements (smiles, hugs, words of praise) were used additionally, as well as more generalized reinforcement. Following appropriate behavior, students were rewarded at the end of lunch by being chosen as line leader or to hold the cafeteria door open or carry the snack box back to their classroom. The use of timeout, ignoring inappropriate behavior and removal of food were also incorporated at mealtime.

During the school year that the therapist worked with this group of children, an improvement in social skills was observed and teaching staff was not as overwhelmed at lunch time. In addition, throughout the school year, children went on field trips within the community and had a chance to practice their new skills at McDonald's and other local restaurants. They were well accepted and always invited back. Carry-over with families was not as successful. Feeding suggestions were sent home periodically, and the therapist was always available at parent meetings and school open houses. However, parent attendance was poor, and it was often found that despite simple suggestions, parents did not spend time to structure or reinforce an appropriate mealtime environment.

SETTING B

This is a public elementary school with a Special Education Wing in which 17 physically handicapped children ages 3–15 years were divided into 2 classes. Diagnoses included cerebral palsy, muscular dystrophy, spina bifida, hearing impaired, and developmentally delayed and the children presented a variety of needs. Evaluation of each child provided the baseline for programming both in individual and group treatment. The occupational therapist was available three times a week at lunch time. In addition to working on proper positioning, use of necessary equipment, and general ability to provide adequate nutrition, the goal of making meal time a fun and pleasureable experience for the students as well as staff was emphasized. Specific physical goals included improving oral-motor development (i.e., sucking, swallowing, decrease drooling, and lip closure), increasing independence in eating (from finger feeding to grasp of spoon, scooping, hand to mouth sequence, and then cup drinking and use of a fork) and training in the use of adaptive equipment.

A team approach with teachers, aides, and volunteers was encouraged to promote normal and independent feeding experiences. The occupational therapist often worked as a consultant to achieve this after evaluating children and initiating programs. All of the children were fed in adaptive chairs (mostly Rifton) except one who was fed in her wheelchair. Adaptive equipment included built-up handle utensils, scoop dishes, plate guards and dycem. Because one of the teachers was trained and certified in neurodevelopmental treatment, she was able to concentrate some on oral facilitation prior to feeding while the occupational therapist worked on positioning at meal time.

Of the group of students who required only consultative services, all were independent using a minimal amount of adaptive equipment. Minimal assistance from their classmates or other schoolmates to open some food containers or cut up some meats was needed. For those children who were seen in a group setting, ongoing progress has been made. Some are now independent with feeding, except for needing help to cut up various foods and for opening milk cartons. Also, they need encouragement to try new foods. Of the remaining children seen, intense individual programming continues with emphasis on improving oral-motor skills. All of the children are required to take at least one bite of everything before they can receive dessert and as best they can, help wipe their hands and face and clean their table area.

SETTING C

Children, aged 1 month–5 years were seen at the day school of a private, non-profit residential and day care facility. Primarily, they were severely physically and mentally handicapped children; some were language delayed and considered as trainable or educable mentally handicapped. Diagnoses included cerebral palsy, failure to thrive, seizure disorders, visual impairments, and agenesis of the corpus collosum. Children were seen for feeding training in two classrooms—one for infants and one for preschoolers, even though a kitchen and small room for occupational therapy are in the building. Meals consist of whatever the cafeteria in the main residence sends over or baby food provided by parents of the day care children. The kitchen in the classroom building has a microwave oven and a food processor which are used as necessary by the occupational therapist. The infants (twelve) are all individually fed except one or two who can be worked with together by one person, and the preschoolers (eight) eat all at one time. In addition to lunch, all infants and preschoolers received a snack in the morning and some of the failure to thrive children were provided with breakfast. Therefore, feeding training was able to take place at any of those times depending on the child's needs and the foods served.

All of the children were evaluated and individualized goals established. The children presented a wide range of feeding problems from having nasogastric tubes, to those just beginning oral feedings, to some who had potential for total independence in eating. Since the teacher and aide in the preschool class were not receptive to change, that group had not had any occupational therapy beyond evaluation at the beginning of the school year. Fortunately, all of these children fed themselves fairly well. It was hoped, however, that after the teacher and aide saw what successes occurred from intervention by the occupational therapist in the infant class they would be more receptive to collaboration for children in the preschool class during the next year.

In the infant group, children were typically fed in travel chairs, infant feeder seats or at a small table. Goals often included helping the teacher with positioning. (Equipment was scarce. Another major goal was to locate funds and equipment.) Since parents in this program were fairly interested, especially in feeding, their participation and observation was encouraged. Many of the parents of the infants came in at least two times during the school year for specific training and advice about feeding techniques. The occupational therapist conducted follow-up with them throughout the year to assure carry-over. In addition, instruction of staff for each child's specific needs was carried out and emphasized.

Due to the infants' schedule, treatment was provided either at breakfast, snack time, or at lunch. The entire feeding time was rarely spent with just one child. Most often, a half hour was split between treatment of two or three children. Emphasis was on initiating programs which could then be carried out by the teacher and aide. They usually followed through with facilitation and positioning but this cooperation took all year to achieve. While carry-over was not always consistent, it did improve. Children with the least complex problems were first to be programmed and treatment was directed to providing proper chairs and proper positioning at the table in order to facilitate independent feeding. Next those children who needed guidance in scooping and in developing hand to mouth patterns were addressed. Breakfast or snack time was usually chosen for working with these children since the teacher and aide were freer to observe then as the therapist established eating routines. For the children with the most severe problems (i.e., tactile sensitivity, deficits in oral-motor control, abnormal reflex development), problem solving sessions were conducted by the therapist with the teacher and aide to develop the most feasible approaches to use.

The teacher and aide in the infant class have demonstrated good carry-over, especially regarding desensitization and oral facilitation before feeding due to their positive effects on the feeding process and decreased time elements involved. They still occasionally were not aware of proper positioning and its influence on eating ability. High chairs are used less frequently in favor of travel chairs and modified sitting devices. In general, because of the increased awareness and availability of equipment, carry-over has been better. Plans for the next school year include individualized charts to be made for each child involved in a feeding program with a picture of their equipment and a brief description of positioning and feeding techniques.

CASE HISTORY RB

RB is an 11 year old female, labeled profoundly mentally handicapped but placed in a trainable mentally handicapped program at her mother's insistence. She is in a public school for mentally handicapped children. RB is severely developmentally delayed, with low muscle tone, wide base gait, very short attention span, and is unresponsive to most people or activities (wanders randomly about room, knocks things off shelves, laughs inappropriately). She does not initiate activities on her own, except to lay down at nap time or reach for juice. She has a severe overbite, scraps food off the spoon with her teeth, and pushes the food to the back of her mouth to swallow. She holds a cup with both hands and then drops it after drinking. Feeding is slow and messy.

RB was referred to occupational therapy to try to increase general skills of daily living, especially feeding which would help her teacher and family enormously. A feeding program was initiated. While RB ate in the classroom with the other children, she was seen individually by the occupational therapist. Feeding training occurred twice a week during the school year for approximately 45 minutes each session. When time allowed, gross motor activities, tactile stimulation and vestibular stimulation were used by the therapist before feeding activities.

Goals were modest in view of RB's limitations, but included: improve muscle tone in oral musculature, increase eye contact with plate, utensils, food and hands, enhance general attention to task and, finally, to encourage appropriate hand to mouth patterns. Strategies included initially providing adaptive equipment (i.e., Rifton chair, scoop dish, built-up handle utensil) and initiating some neurodevelopmental treatment techniques, especially in regard to positioning. Any beverage, especially juice, was a motivation and reward for RB during actual training. Physical assistance, verbal commands, and positive and negative reinforcement were also consistently used. Ongoing consultation with mother and teacher was made to reinforce skills. Mother came in seven times during the school year and provided good follow-through at home.

At the end of the school year, RB exhibited progress, especially in improved muscle tone. Her sitting posture improved by use of her adaptive chair. Better positioning and posture led to improved lip closure, thus decreasing drooling and increasing her ability to scoop food off utensils with her lips. Chewing and swallowing improved as well. Although her grasp remained weak, RB spontaneously reached for and grasped a spoon, fork and cup. Built-up handles were decreased in size twice during the year.

Eye contact, attention to task, and hand to mouth patterns improved, although feeding continued to be messy. Grabbing food decreased significantly and stopped quickly with only verbal reminders. RB kept her hands on the table without any reminders. She scooped food but did not look at what she was doing. Motions remained uncoordinated when bringing the spoon or fork to her mouth. RB was able to lower her cup to the table but this too was done in an uncoordinated manner. Unless reminded, she would frequently drop it.

Overall progress was attributed to the fact that RB was seen individually for feeding training with good classroom and home carry-over. By first addressing basic positioning needs, a sound foundation was established on which RB could feel secure, receive positive feedback and begin to be successful in general feeding skills. Simple and consistent verbal and physical commands and cues encouraged further reinforcement.

SUMMARY AND CONCLUSIONS

Feeding problems of the multi-handicapped child have been recognized and dealt with as part of the scope of occupational therapy. The itinerant occupational therapist in a county school program finds herself addressing issues beyond the immediate feeding difficulties presented. Therapists are faced with high caseloads and limited time available in their treatment schedules. Additionally, school personnel are confronted with increased numbers in the classroom, more complex feeding problems to work with and a lower staff-to-student ratio. As each school year begins, therapists need to quickly assess the situations at feeding times.

Positioning and equipment needs should be addressed as early as possible. This not only benefits the student but helps the classroom staff by ultimately making their involvement at mealtime easier and faster. If this is achieved early on, the rapport established between the classroom staff and occupational therapist can be a positive foundation for the more involved feeding skills to be taught and carried out later. While providing adaptive equipment is usually essential, it is important to keep it minimal and simple so as not to overwhelm the student and staff. Once these basic needs are met successfully, additional feeding skills can be emphasized. The occupational therapist then can evaluate which students would benefit most from direct services when time permits or how to best utilize her time providing consultative services.

The programs and case history described were intended to give an overview of feeding problems seen in schools where multi-handicapped children are served. Further it was shown how they have been met by itinerant occupational therapists who have infrequent but on-going contact with both students and staff. Because therapist time is so limited, rapport with school staff is extremely important for program follow-up. Each child's needs must be evaluated, prioritized, and broken down into achievable goals. Only then can all involved feel successful.

Systems Theory and Feeding Programs: Application in a Mental Retardation Institution

Beverley J. Gaines, MS, OTR, FAOTA

ABSTRACT. Eating, as one of the basic processes of life, is a skill vulnerable to disruption from a wide variety of insults. The typical mental retardation institution with residents of many age and ability levels provides a spectrum of eating/feeding disorders. The institution also includes many service systems which interact to provide mealtime services. These include training programs, direct care, dietary, and medical-nursing services.

This paper describes the development of a complex, comprehensive feeding program in a 120-bed mental retardation institution. Components of the program include staff training, diagnostic and diet clinics, evaluation and resident training, and dining room management. The application of General Systems Theory to the feeding program is described and implications for the development of similar programs are discussed.

Eating is an activity universally engaged in by all ages and conditions of persons. Yet, it is an activity composed of many acquired skills ranging from mastication to manners. As such, it is an activity peculiarly vulnerable to disruptions from a diverse array

---

Beverley J. Gaines is co-founder of ADAPT/ABILITY, Inc., and has a private practice in Asheville, NC, in addition to part-time employment at Black Mountain Center, near Asheville. Material for this paper was gathered from experience at the Black Mountain Center, where she has been lead occupational therapist since 1980. Portions of this material have been presented to conferences of AOTA, NCOTA, NC-AAMD, and Mountain Area Health Education Center (MAHEC) in Asheville. The author is grateful for the working relationship with all the staff at the Black Mountain Center, which enabled this program to develop and continue. Special recognition is extended to LeAnn Martin, CCC-Sp, and Suzanne Balboni-Kielbasa, Staff Development Specialist, for their roles in the initial development of the program.

This article appears jointly in *Occupational Therapy for People With Eating Dysfunctions* (The Haworth Press, Inc., 1986) and *Occupational Therapy in Health Care*, Volume 3, Number 2 (Summer 1986).

101

of insults—ranging from delayed development to disordered social interaction.

A mental retardation institution is a microcosm of the myriad of disorders that can disrupt eating. Typically, the residents exhibit a wide range of disability from profound retardation and severe neuromuscular disorders to mild retardation characterized by social ineptitude. Thus, the mental retardation institution offers an ideal situation for the study and correction of eating problems. Additionally, a mental retardation institution allows a study of the interaction between management systems and human needs systems.

This paper describes the development of a complex and comprehensive feeding program in a small mental retardation institution. The evolving course of the program over a five-year period demonstrates responses to predictable phenomena of General Systems Theory. The paper will describe the development of the Feeding Program, pertinent components of General Systems Theory with specific Feeding Program examples, and implications for future development of institution based feeding programs.

SETTING FOR THE FEEDING PROGRAM

Black Mountain Center (BMC) is a 120-bed mental retardation institution localed in Western North Carolina. It was established in 1977 to relieve crowding at other centers and to allow residents to be nearer their families. For its first five years, it functioned administratively as a satellite unit of an older institution 50 miles away and was dependent on the parent institution for financial resources and resolution of major management problems. Two management concerns relevant to this paper were (1) the conversion of a 600-bed tuberculosis sanatorium into an appropriate physical plant for mental retardation and (2) retraining of sanatorium staff to work with the mentally retarded.

The 120 residents at BMC represent a wide range of age and ability. Approximately two-thirds are non-ambulatory. Developmental skills range from one month to 5 years, averaging between 15 and 18 months. The chronological age range is 5–62 years, with a mean age range of 27–35 years. Many residents have been institutionalized for twenty years or longer. The residents live in three units of 40 residents each with placement generally along skill levels. Each of the three units has its own "speciality staff", including occupational, physical and speech therapists; educators, recreators, psychologist and social worker. Speciality staff include technicians assigned to work with professional staff; in most instances, technicians have practical experience but little formal training in the speciality area.

ORGANIZATION OF THE FEEDING PROGRAM

In 1980, a Dining Task Force was appointed by the Executive Committee to study the quality of life in dining at Black Mountain Center. Although this Task Force completed its mission and was dissolved in 1981 after approximately 9 months of work, the mealtime program at BMC has continued and become both complex and comprehensive. The following description will present the current organization as well as some of the relevant historical development. Dates for start-up of each component are noted in parentheses. The reader will note that historical development and logical organization are not always parallel!

Dining Task Force (Fall 1980–Summer 1981)

The Dining Task Force was created by the Executive Committee to improve the dining situation and to correct an ICF survey deficiency. The Task Force was interdisciplinary being chaired by the Speech Pathologist. Other members included a COTA, Dietitian, and unit representatives. (When first appointed, there was not a full-time OTR at BMC; after the author's arrival, occupational therapy input was doubled to this committee.)

In 1980, residents were fed in dayrooms by direct care staff. The reader will recall that residents had been transferred (usually in groups of ten or twenty) from other institutions which were overcrowded. As a consequence of the overcrowding and understaffing, many residents had grossly inadequate feeding skills and poor nutritional status. The majority of direct care staff had transferred from the sanatorium and had little prior experience with the mentally retarded. In addition, positions at state institutions were being cut due to the economic recession of the early '80's.

The Dining Task Force studied all areas of feeding from staffing patterns, possible space for dining rooms, and training needs to equipment needs, taste and consistency of food, and dining atmosphere. As a result of their study, two indepth workshops on feeding techniques were offered to staff; three dining rooms were created; staffing patterns and scheduling were altered and new responsibilities were assigned to many staff.

Although the Task Force was dissolved in 1981, a lasting legacy was created to emphasize the importance of feeding as a major event and skill area in the lives of the residents.

Goals and Policies

The three major goals defined by the Dining Task Force have continued as the foundation for all future developments in the Feeding Program. These goals are:

1. To provide sound nutrition to all residents
2. To provide a normalized dining atmosphere (this includes space, decor, time allowance, noise levels, and staff attitudes)
3. To provide learning opportunities at all levels of development.

In further support of these goals, a policy was established by Executive Committee that each staff member who would be feeding residents must have formal feeding training before being assigned to feeding duties. Job descriptions of speciality staff were broadened to include feeding two meals per day.

Management Support

On the whole, top management has been supportive of all feeding programs. This has included establishment of the Task Force; re-allocating time, resources and manpower to create dining rooms; setting policies, and negotiating schedules. In retrospect, an error was made when dissolving the Task Force in not delegating follow-up responsibility as a structural task—i.e., on an organization chart or job description. While management did support feeding programs, the major focus of management attention for nearly two years was the effort to gain independent status for BMC. As a result, other program priorities were established without clearly examining how they would affect the quality of feeding. This was also a period of massive staff turnover with a loss of training skills and enthusiasm. Attention was recaptured in December, 1983 by assertive action from occupational therapy (described later) and currently a high level of management support is present.

Dining Needs Committee (1984)

In June, 1984 a Dining Needs Committee was formally sanctioned by the Executive Committee with the chairperson designated to be the Lead Occupational Therapist. The purpose of the committee is to oversee and coordinate all feeding related activities, to make recommendations as needed to management, and to implement changes. The committee began with a list of 23 areas of concerns, compiled by the lead occupational therapist, and by summer, 1985, had whittled the list down to about three areas.

Following BMC tradition, membership on the committee is representative of many professional areas and levels of employment. Membership is stipulated to include the dietitian, advocate, staff development specialist, and unit representation. Current unit representation includes speech pathologist, recreation therapist, vocational educator, a COTA, an education assistant, and a developmental technician supervisor.

The structural components and programs under the overall supervision of the Dining Needs Committee are described below.

Feeding Training (1981)

Feeding Training was the earliest mandated ongoing activity of the Feeding Program. Initially devised by the Lead Speech Pathologist (and chair of the Dining Task Force), the Lead Occupational Therapist, and a Staff Development Specialist, the training was a day-long instructional session. At its onset, feeding training was presented bi-monthly to groups of 15–20 staff until all staff had been trained. Thereafter, it has been regularly given on a monthly basis to new employees. On several occasions, shortened versions have been given to groups of student nurses or volunteers. In summer, 1985, a special session was given for Executive Committee as a group.

While the format for training has changed several times, content is essentially the same as originally designed. Currently, training is held the third day of the month (all employees now report on the first day of the month). Supervised experience in feeding follows the designated instruction.

Since 1981 several hundred persons have been trained as feeders. The list includes all developmental technicians, RN's, LPN's, all speciality staff, advocates, staff development personnel, chaplain, lab and x-ray technologists, dietitians, Executive Committee, and some clerical staff. Students, volunteers, and CETA workers go through training. Occupational therapy students on affiliation attend class the first month and subsequently assist in teaching the class.

Dining Room Coordinators (1982) and Supervisors (1984)

In 1982 the Executive Committee agreed to allow release time to staff members to serve as coordinators for the unit dining rooms. The duties of the coordinator were to ensure smooth running of the Unit Dining Room by supervising the feeders, monitoring diet trays, and seeing that linens and supplies were available. The role of the Dining Room Coordinator was seen differently by each unit and consequently the daily quality control was dependent upon each unit's perception of the role. This was one of the major concerns studied by the Dining Needs Committee. In 1984, management agreed to the following role definitions:

1. The Dining Room Coordinator (DRC) would be either the OTR or COTA on the unit. The DRC would be responsible for doing feeding evaluations, writing feeding guidelines and programs, training new staff, and acquiring special feeding equipment. The DRC usually does intensive feeding training with hard-to-feed residents and then trains other staff to take over.
2. A new post, Dining Room Supervisor, would be filled from unit staff chosen on the basis of competence, interest, and rapport with staff. The specific responsibilities of the supervisor are to see that the Dining Room is properly set up, to assign staff to feed residents, monitor diet trays, and monitor staff performance. If the supervisor is absent, the DRC acts as supervisor or delegates duties.

In practice, the Coordinators and Supervisors work closely together to devise feeding groupings and monitor all aspects of feeding. The Coordinators and Supervisors are members of the Dining Needs Committee, and thus are aware of problems and solutions in other dining rooms.

Unit Dining Management Teams (1981)

Composition of these teams has varied over time and according to unit priorities. Teams meet as needed to work on management problems which may range from "housekeeping is not stocking the closet" to "that employee has a bad attitude." Teams usually consist of the coordinator (OTR) and Dining Room Supervisor and perhaps include the unit manager or R.N.

Feeding Clinic (1981)

The concept and format of feeding clinic was devised in 1981 to provide a more complex evaluation of feeding behavior when needed with specific residents. Feeding Clinic is held on an as-needed basis and chaired by the unit OTR or COTA. Other staff are requested to attend according to the residents' needs. The primary feeder and the advocate always attend. Others may be the dietitian, R.N., psychologist or other staff. Each participant is expected to become familiar with the resident's feeding problem before the clinic date. The clinic itself provides a means to experiment with different feeding techniques, to observe staff-resident interaction, or sometimes to discuss possible outcomes and strategies. Originally, each participant submitted a short report; these were compiled into a report and co-signed by all. Since 1984, the occupational therapist has written the report, incorporating all input, but organizing the report to correspond with the AOTA Uniform Terminology. All participants still co-sign, as well as the supervising OTR, if the clinic was chaired by a COTA.

Occupational therapy is responsible for follow-up from clinics and for seeing that recommendations are distributed to appropriate persons.

Diet Clinic (1983)

Diet Clinic was organized on one unit as a pilot project and since has been instituted on other units in a modified form. Diet Clinic focuses on nutritional issues, weight gain/loss, food preferences, and general health. The Clinic is chaired by the DRC/OT and other participants include M.D., R.N., dietitian, advocate, and dining room supervisor. Occasionally, the pharmacist will be asked to attend, if a drug interaction is at question. Typically, five to eight residents will be discussed. Clinic is held once or twice monthly.

Minutes are circulated to all unit staff and each discussion is recorded as a ''mini-team'' in the resident's chart.

THE FEEDING PROGRAM AS AN EXAMPLE OF SYSTEMS THEORY

About two years after the initial formation of the original Dining Task Force, the relevance of systems theory to the developing Feeding Program was noted. From that time forward, a conscious effort was made to apply systems theory concepts to the Feeding Program, a decision that enabled future development to occur more logically.

Characteristics of Systems

Systems theory hypothesizes that all endeavors are characterized by certain basic processes, the sum of which can be categorized as a ''system.'' The basic processes include:

1. An identified outcome or product and the marshalling of resources to achieve that outcome.
2. Articulated goals, with policies, operating procedures, job descriptions, staff roles and functions planned to achieve the outcome.
3. Interaction between components of the system.
4. Continuous information flow between internal components as well as between the system and external environment.
5. Responsiveness and a means of correction or monitoring action to correspond with information from other sources. This may even include alteration of desired outcomes into another form.

A system usually does not operate in isolation, but rather in interaction with other systems. In addition, very often a system is itself comprised of several ''sub-systems''. Interaction between either sub-systems or entire systems may be visualized as occurring on either a horizontal plane or on a vertical plane. For example, within a hospital there may be more or less horizontal systems of laboratory services, clerical services, and dietary services. On the other hand, there is usually a vertical system of human needs—thus lab and dietary services will receive far more financial support than library and recreation services which are usually provided by volunteers.

Certain dynamic principles govern the interaction of sub-systems or multiple systems. These include:

1. An area of shared responsibilities, concern, and possible friction where the systems interact. In actual practice, these areas may seem inconsequential but consume enormous amounts of time to keep operating smoothly.
2. A system constantly seeks to keep itself in equilibrium by making continual internal adjustments in response to external forces. In a complex organization with many sub-systems operating both vertically and horizontally the number of internal adjustments being continually made is almost overwhelming. If at the same time the organization itself is attempting to maintain equilibrium in the "outside system", e.g., the business world, the political system—then there is an increased possibility that actions within the sub-systems are not going to mesh with larger goals.
3. The alerting mechanism of a system will be diverted to new developments and information, thereby requiring an already functioning sub-system to enhance its distress signal when dysfunctioning. In other words, "the wheel that squeaks the loudest gets the most grease."
4. In a functional system, one information point will emerge as the pivot around which all other components will eventually oscillate. In today's jargon, this is often called the "bottom line."

The Feeding Program as a System and a Sub-System

The Feeding Program at BMC functions as a system with identified goals, procedures, roles and functions of participants, and interacting components. It has at least two identifiable sub-systems within itself—a training sub-system and a service-delivery system. As a service-delivery system it interacts horizontally with other service delivery systems, and as such, there are identifiable inter-action/friction areas. Two examples will illustrate this principle: (1) In the area of scheduling, the basic care and hygiene requirements continuously conflict with meal times. On days when a unit is short-staffed, there must be adjustment of scheduling for feeding, bathing and toileting, and off-unit programming. (2) Certain subsidiary needs always seem to be "somebody else's job." For example, whose job is it to stock the Dining Room linen closet? Does this belong to housekeeping, to the Dining Room Supervisor, or to individual feeding staff? Or, is it a task that can be assumed by a resident on Internal Placement Job Training? The reader can no doubt think of numerous similar examples in which enormous amounts of time have never led to any lasting solution.

The Feeding Program also can be seen to interact in a vertical manner with other systems. As a service delivery system it has achieved a lasting place because it satisfies basic biological needs. As such, feeding has precedence over educational programming, a ranking which periodically causes great resentment among all specialty staff other than occupational therapists. Interestingly within the Feeding Program itself, there is a continual preoccupation with the oral-motor and dietary aspects to the subordination of the social aspects, thus further illustrating the point that basic needs must be satisfied first.

While the Feeding program has a solid acceptance as a system to satisfy the basic needs of residents, it is only one system within BMC. Similarly, BMC itself is only a sub-system within the Department of Human Resources of the State of North Carolina. This became painfully obvious when BMC was in the process of seeking independent status as a state agency. For approximately 18 months, the attention of top management was almost totally diverted to interaction with external systems. Internal systems were assumed to be functional and only cursory attention was given to the interaction of these internal systems. Assignment of priorities to staff and projects was done on the basis of external forces, such as accrediting agencies, with little attention to effects on already existing programs. In reference to the Feeding Program, the Dining Task Force had been dissolved and no person or group was designated as responsible for its quality. An external monitoring system, devised to meet accreditation standards, began monitoring all aspects of staff performance. The result was that although staff were cited for inadequate feeding techniques, no mechanism (other than disciplinary action) was available to place responsibility or to provide corrective action. Predictably, inordinate amounts of time were spent trying to comply with the monitoring system where a more direct and efficient solution would have been a structural assignment of responsibility for this particular outcome. It was during this period that the author really became aware of Systems Theory as a reality, rather than an abstraction.

The Feeding Program: Communications Methods in the System

Once identified as a system, communication methods were seen as a major component of the Feeding Program. These methods take several forms.

1. The same knowledge base is made available to all staff via Feeding Training. Regardless of former experience, all new employees are required to go through training, so that they are aware of what their colleagues have been exposed to. Furthermore, the knowledge base has been put into a fairly standardized form so that it is not dependent on only one person to transmit it.

2. Findings on individual residents are documented in the Unit Chart, available to all staff. Specific techniques and procedures are made available in the Dining Room via Feeding Guideline Cards. In addition, a dietary card accompanies each tray at each meal, so that contents may be quickly checked against dietary requirements.

3. Minutes of management meetings are circulated to all unit staff with copies going to top management and advocacy. Dining Needs Committee minutes are circulated to all unit managers and top management, to the members who represent each unit and all pertinent departments.

4. Access to management is available via minutes distribution, plus an automatic request to appear in person at Executive Committee when any recommendation is made which requires Executive action. There is also quarterly access to management with less pressing problems via regular meetings between the lead occupational therapist and the Director of Program Services.

5. Direct supervision and modeling of techniques occur on a daily basis as the Dining Room Coordinator also feeds at each meal.

6. As a sub-system of both Feeding Program and Staff Development, the Feeding Training can easily be expanded to provide information on new techniques. Currently, new staff

training is being planned to include specific training on aspiration problems and on video fluorographic swallow studies, a newly diagnostic tool in the community. Staff targeted for these presentations will be physicians, nurses, speech pathologists, and Dining Room Supervisors. This training was requested by Dietary and Occupational Therapy, both departments having received training at the local Area Health Education Center (AHEC).

7. An informal communication network on feeding problems exists externally to BMC organized through the Allied Health Programs at AHEC. This is currently allowing comparison of swallow studies on mentally retarded persons with those done on victims of head-trauma, CVA, and cancer.

The Feeding Program: Identifying the Pivotal Point

Throughout the history of the Feeding Program, and in fact, pre-dating it, one component always remained in place—the Dietary Card. No matter what disaster might occur during mealtime, the Diet Cards were always carefully retrieved and returned to their file box on the food cart for use at the next meal.

The Diet Cards at BMC are 5 × 8 file cards, containing resident's name and color-coded dietary instructions for diet consistency, listing of food dislikes, and any special information such as low-sodium, counted calories, added bran, double servings, etc.

When it was realized that only the Diet Cards had not changed, it then became obvious that nutrition was the basic area of data that had to be monitored. The pivotal point then was identified as the Ideal Body Weight (IBW), a range of 8–10 pounds considered as ideal for a person's age, height, sex, and body build.

Following identification of the IBW as the key indicator for all other feeding data, the Diet Clinic was established on a pilot basis. The IBW has continued to be a reliable correlate of all feeding problems, whether behavioral, nutritional, or medical.

IMPLICATIONS FOR SIMILAR PROGRAMS

Will It Work Here?

Institutional size and organizational structure and goals will determine whether a feeding program of such complexity is appropriate. Certain characteristics would seem transferable to most situations. These are: a training component for staff, a means for evaluating results and instituting changes, a method of communicating, a person or committee clearly designated to be responsible and accountable.

What's the Pay-Off?

The results at BMC clearly indicate the effort is worthwhile. In 1980, the two non-ambulatory units had no more than 6 self-feeders among the 80 residents. That number has now increased to nearly 40 in addition to 4 residents placed elsewhere. Average length of time to feed specific residents has decreased dramatically, in one instance from 1 hour 20 minutes to 25 minutes. Several residents who once were automatically assigned to the occupational therapist as difficult to feed, are now considered "easy" and can be fed by almost anyone. One resident has progressed completely off gastrostomy feeding, and no resident is totally fed by gastrostomy. Most residents are within IBW range, although there are usually 3 or 4 who are being monitored.

From the staff standpoint, team interaction is greatly increased, as is respect for professional expertise in other fields. Also, at least 3 staff have been able to apply feeding skills with their seriously ill family members.

Can One Person Beat the System?

Experience at BMC indicates that if an individual is aware of systems, then that person can work *with* the system to bring about changes. Knowledge of system dynamics is vital to causing a change.

The Feeding Program at BMC got its start from a concerned speech pathologist who was subsequently appointed Task Force Chairperson. Feeding Training was instigated through the remark of the occupational therapist to the Executive Committee. At times, the need for one person to initiate action is definitely risk-taking, as when the lead occupational therapist compiled a list of 23 problem areas—many of them of a managerial nature.

Perhaps the most important lessons learned from the Feeding Program at BMC are these:

1. Be confident of your professional expertise but not jealous of your territory.
2. Preoccupation by management with a larger task does not necessarily mean that management is against your program.
3. In setting up a program of any kind, a way must be found to ensure continuity of the program, independent of the individual persons involved.
4. Changing a method or procedure to be more responsive to a need is a necessity to keep a program relevant and feasible.
5. The sooner you can identify your key indicator or "bottom line", the more quickly your program will gain legitimacy with other staff.
6. True, but often overlooked, is that you learn from both negative and positive results. Instead of being defeated by a bad results, analyze it to find how it can be turned to better advantage.

SUMMARY

The experience of the author in developing and maintaining a complex Feeding Program demonstrate that on-going management of a service program is enhanced by knowledge and conscious application of system theory. Awareness of the dynamics in systems theory will allow identification of conflict areas and aid in obtaining favorable allocations of resources. Finally, awareness of systems theory enables an individual to influence the functioning of a system in a long-lasting manner.

REFERENCES

1. Cohen M A, Gross P J: The Developmental Resource: Behavioral Sequences for Assessment and Program Planning. Vol. I. New York: Grune and Stratton. 1979. Pp. 159–182

2. Gallender D: Eating Handicaps: Illustrated Techniques for Feeding Disorders. Springfield, Il: Charles C. Thomas, Publisher. 1979.

3. Korabek C A, Reid D H, Ivancic M T: Improving needed food intake of profoundly handicapped children through effective supervision of institutional staff. *App Res in Men Ret*, 2: 69–88, 1981

4. Lazlo E: The Systems View of the World. New York: Braziller, 1974

5. Mann W C, Sobset R: Feeding programs for the institutionalized mentally retarded. *Am J of Occ Ther* 29: 79–85, 1978

6. Morris, S E: Program Guidelines for Children with Feeding Problems. Edison, N.J.: Childcraft Education Corporation, 1977

7. Perske R, Clifton A, McLean B M, Stein J J (eds.): Mealtimes for Severely and Profoundly Handicapped Persons. Baltimore: University Park Press, 1977

8. Schaefer M: Administration of Environmental Health Programmes: a Systems View. Geneva: World Health Organization, 1974

9. Springer N S: Nutrition Casebook on Developmental Disabilities. Syracuse, N.Y.: Syracuse University Press, 1982

10. Stratton M: Behavioral assessment scale of oral functions in feeding. *Am J of Occ Ther* 35: 719–721, 1981

11. Wilson J (ed): Oral-Motor Function and Dysfunction in Children. Chapel Hill, N.C.: Univ. of North Carolina, Div. of Physical Therapy, 1977

RELATED READINGS

Adams J L: Conceptual Blockbusting: a Pleasureable Guide to Better Problem Solving. New York: W W Norton, 1974. Chap. 4 "Emotional Blocks"

Davis R H, Alexander L T, Yelon S L: Learning System Design. New York: McGraw-Hill, 1974

Mager R F, Pipe P: Analyzing Performance Problems: or "You Really Oughta Wanna". Belmont, CA: Fearon Pub., 1970

Mager R F, Beach K M: Developing Vocational Instruction. Belmont, CA: Fearon Pub., 1967

Morris S E: The Normal Acquisition of Oral Feeding Skills: Implications for Assessment and Treatment. New York: Therapeutic Media, Inc., 1982

Netter F H: The Digestive System, Part I. Vol. 3 of the CIBA Collection of Medical Illustrations. Summit, NJ: CIBA Pharmaceutical Co.

Utley B L, Helvoet J R, Barnes K: Handling, Positioning, and Feeding the Physically Handicapped. In Educational Programming for the Severely/Profoundly Handicapped. Sontag E, Smith J, Certo N (eds): Reston, VA: CEC, 1977

Zinkus C: Feeding Skill Training. In Feeding the Handicapped Child, MAH Smith (ed.) Memphis, TN: Child Development Center. 1969

PRACTICE WATCH: THINGS TO THINK ABOUT

"In Search of Excellence"— Professional Parallels to a Business Orientation

Helen M. Madill, PhD, OT(C)
E. Sharon Brintnell, BOT, MSc, OT(C)
Rita den Otter, BSc, OT(C)

ABSTRACT. Peters and Waterman (1983) have reviewed and profiled some of America's leading corporations, in order to determine what might account for their success. This paper reviews Peters' and Waterman's basic tenets and draws parallels for occupational therapy. The outcome of their comprehensive review of management practices is applied to occupational therapy. Recent research is used to support these contentions and recommendations for action on a departmental or unit level are discussed.

Helen M. Madill is Associate Professor, and E. Sharon Brintnell is Chairman and Associate Professor, in the Department of Occupational Therapy at the University of Alberta, Edmonton, Alberta, Canada. Rita den Otter is Director of Occupational Therapy at the University of Alberta Hospitals, Edmonton, Alberta, Canada.

The assistance of Drs. L. L. Stewin, G. W. Fitzsimmons, and D. Macnab with the Canadian study is gratefully acknowledged.

This article appears jointly in *Occupational Therapy for People With Eating Dysfunctions* (The Haworth Press, Inc., 1986) and *Occupational Therapy in Health Care*, Volume 3 Number 2 (Summer 1986).

117

As the economics of health care become an ever increasing cost burden and a public issue, both institutions and governments search for better methods of cost control. To do this, an increasing number of institutions are turning to business and commerce, implementing administrative models that are more typical of the corporate structure. The chief executive officer of many hospitals is now frequently called the president; vice-presidents have replaced the more familiar heads of services and strategic planning must be more closely related to the health of the operating budget. In Canada some ministers of health have stated that they would like to see private enterprise run a medical facility on an experimental basis, so that cost comparisons could be made.

These changes have implications for the services offered by such units as occupational therapy. It may represent the inevitable scenario to some therapists, progress or even commercialization to others. Whatever one's attitude, as a therapist the corporate model will influence the profession's practice models throughout the coming decades.

Peters and Waterman in their book "In Search of Excellence" reviewed and profiled some of America's leading corporations in order to determine what might account for their success. The outcome of their comprehensive review of management practices can be applied to occupational therapy unit management and service delivery. This paper will review Peters and Waterman's major tenets and draw parallels for occupational therapy. Recent research will be used to support these contentions and recommendations for action on a departmental or unit level will be discussed.

Peters and Waterman[1] considered seven primary variables and treated them as interdependent when conducting their review; these included: "structure, strategy, people, management style, systems and procedures, guiding concepts and shared values (i.e., culture), and the present and hoped for corporate strengths or skills" (p.9). This they organized into what became known as the "McKinsey 7-S Framework". Shared values form the hub of the hexagonal model.

This central element, surrounded by and interconnected with strategy and structure, is described as the hardware of the organization. Systems, style, staff and skills are the remaining software components. If shared values comprise the central element in this model, what is known about the values held by occupational therapists?

Canadian study data from a sample of occupational therapists in

Canada (N = 1400) provided information about their values.[2] With over 50% representation of occupational therapists from each region of the country it is possible to consider the findings from the survey as relatively representative of the total population.

The Life Roles Inventory,[3,4] later referred to as the LRI, was used in this national survey. The LRI is a self administered vocationally related inventory with two major sections: a values inventory which measures the importance of specific values, and a salience inventory that measures the importance of specific roles.[5] In terms of values, respondents are asked to indicate the degree of importance they attach to 100 statements on a four-point Likert-type scale. Each of the statements has been assigned to one of twenty value scales (e.g., achievement, altruism, autonomy, etc.). The salience inventory has the respondent focus on five key activities: studying, working, community service, home/family and leisure. The level of participation (amount of time spent), commitment (feelings about) and role values that the respondent seeks is again measured on a four point scale under each of the five key activities.

Coefficient alpha interval consistency reliabilities have been completed for each value scale. Reliability coefficients range from 0.72–0.86 with a median of 0.80. Internal consistency coefficients for participation range from 0.85–0.95, commitment 0.89–0.95 and for role values 0.87–0.90. An acceptable level of concurrent validity was demonstrated between the LRI and three major vocational inventories.

As outlined in Figure 1, occupational therapist (N = 1400) endorsed the twenty values from the LRI at the levels reported below.

VALUES

Further analysis of the data presented in Figure 1 according to age, position category (staff therapists, supervisor, private practitioner) and respondents' highest educational level, indicated that occupational therapists in Canada endorse the same values. Homogeneity is observed in the six highest value scale ratings endorsed across all classification variables: personal development, ability utilization, social relations, achievement, altruism, autonomy, occur in that order. Only in the case of those with doctoral degrees

FIGURE 1

LRI VALUE SCALE RATINGS,
MEANS AND STANDARD DEVIATIONS

VALUES   VALUE SCALE RATINGS

VALUES	$\bar{X}$	SD	1	2	3	4
Ability-Utilization	3.4	0.4				
Achievement	3.3	0.4				
Advancement	2.7	0.6				
Aesthetics	2.6	0.7				
Altruism	3.3	0.5				
Authority	2.9	0.6				
Autonomy	3.3	015				
Creativity	3.2	0.6				
Economics	3.0	0.6				
Life Style	3.0	0.5				
Personal Development	3.6	0.3				
Physical Activity	2.8	0.6				
Prestige	3.0	0.6				
Risk	1.8	0.6				
Social Interaction	2.9	0.6				
Social Relations	3.4	0.5				
Variety	2.9	0.6				
Working Conditions	2.8	0.6				
Cultural Identity	2.6	0.6				
Physical Prowess	1.6	0.6				

1 = Little or no importance
2 = Some importance
3 = Important
4 = Very important

(N = 7) does the rating given to autonomy surpass that assigned to personal development.

The value scales that are of least importance also remain the same: physical prowess and risk. Cultural identity, aesthetics, advancement, physical activity and working conditions are of some importance to therapists but those values are consistently included in six value scales that receive the lowest ratings.

By examining these data one can see that occupational therapists value their contribution to society highly; they strongly endorse helping others and looking after their welfare. They place a great deal of importance upon developing and using their abilities and skills for this purpose. They do not value the entrepreneurial focus common within the business community, where one would expect to see greater emphasis placed upon risk, advancement and economics.

SALIENCE

To complete the picture one must also ascertain to what extent these occupational therapists seek to implement their role values through their working role. Figure 2 outlines the level of participation, commitment and role value assigned to the five major life roles included on the LRI by occupational therapists (N = 1400).

From Figure 2 it can be seen that occupational therapists participate most extensively in the working role. However, they are equally committed to the working and home/family roles and seek to implement their role values primarily through the home/family and working roles.

FIGURE 2

LRI SALIENCE INVENTORY RATINGS,
MEANS AND STANDARD DEVIATIONS

ROLE PARTICIPATION	$\bar{X}$	SD	1	2	3	4
Studying	2.5	0.7			■	
Working	3.0	0.6			■	
Community Service	1.9	0.7		■		
Home/Family	2.7	0.7			■	
Leisure	2.7	0.6			■	
COMMITMENT						
Studying	2.7	0.7			■	
Working	3.4	0.5				■
Community Service	2.4	0.8		■		
Home/Family	3.4	0.7				■
	2.9	0.6			■	
ROLE VALUE REALIZATION						
Studying	2.5	0.7			■	
Working	3.1	0.5				■
Community Service	2.3	0.7		■		
Home/Family	3.2	0.6				■
Leisure	2.9	0.6			■	
			1	2	3	4

1 = Little or no importance
2 = Some importance
3 = Important
4 = Very important

The working role is important to occupational therapists but their commitment and role value scale responses demonstrate that the home/family role is of equal importance. The competition between these two role demands likely creates individual difficulties that will be dealt with in subsequent publications.

APPLICATIONS TO OCCUPATIONAL THERAPY

It has been established that occupational therapists share the same values and that the working role is important to them. The eight attributes that Peters and Waterman[1] describe as characteristic of successful, innovative companies can now be reviewed and discussed as they apply to the management of occupational therapy units.

1. "*A bias for action*: a preference for doing something—anything—rather than sending a question through cycles and cycles of analyses and committee reports."[1(p.1)]

Occupational therapy is a pragmatic profession; therapists like to get on with the job. Those in clincial settings are faced with challenges/problems that are often unique, as exemplified by a case load of clients/patients each with a specific individual need. The decision making cycle in many large health care facilities likely resembles the recycling process described by Peters and Waterman. Occupational therapy units, however, are much smaller so that this does not become an intra-unit problem, but it may well be an inter-unit difficulty.

All staff have a responsibility for the success of their unit in the wider arena. Together they can problem solve or brainstorm in a manner that will support their leader in his/her negotiation at the middle management level. All too frequently though, supervisors tend to act in isolation, relying on an external locus of control to explain their apparent inability to act effectively. By not giving staff therapists the opportunity to contribute, they effectively negate the value of input from service provider level and send those therapists a powerful message—"Your opinion does not count". If one were to borrow from Peters and Waterman's suggestion of small teams used to test out ideas over comparatively short periods of time, the task force method may assist occupational therapy units to broaden their options and develop their strategies.

2. *"Staying close to the customer*—learning his preferences and catering to them."[1(p.1)]

Peters and Waterman point to the necessity for service providers to listen, intently and regularly. Although occupational therapists pride themselves on their ability to deal with the whole patient, when staff shortages increase case loads, checking the client's level of satisfaction may have low priority. A short, simply constructed questionnaire sent to a random selection of discharged patients on a regular basis, as part of the ongoing administration of the department, could provide valuable information. Not only will it assist the department to improve areas of service but it will also help staff determine what they do well and may be of assistance when justifications for budget submissions are required.

3. *"Autonomy and entrepreneurship*—breaking the corporation into small companies and encouraging them to think independently and competitively."[1(p.1)]

Leaders and innovators are fostered by an organizational structure that allows for creativity and "practical risk taking". Companies using such a strategy "support good tries".

Occupational therapists have been schooled in the team concept so that very few dare to compete, or risk the negative reaction from peers which may result from their entrepreneurial endeavours. Canada's best example of the entrepreneurial spirit in occupational therapy is Community Occupational Therapy Associates (COTA) of Toronto.[7] This group has successfully sought occupational therapy contracts for previously unserviced areas. Groups in other provinces have since followed their enterprising lead.

As the corporate model takes over the major health care facility, the demand for the entrepreneur in the leadership role will increase. Departments must ensure that they foster, as opposed to suppress, those at the staff therapist level who exhibit good leadership/ entrepreneurial skills. Department heads must be careful to marshal their talents, rather than calmly watch high achievers opt to pursue careers in allied fields.

4. *"Productivity through people*—creating in *all* employees the awareness that their best efforts are essential and that they will share in the rewards of the company's success."[1(p.1)]

In successful enterprises the we/they attitude is missing. Productivity depends upon people, front line service personnel in particular, and they deserve as much respect as therapists pay to their client/patient. New ideas may come from many sources within the occupational therapy staff and administrative problem solving must begin with those who will be required to make the system work. Units work better when the staff who are expected to work within the policies or guidelines also have a hand in designing and implementing them.

5. *"Hands-on value driven*—insisting that executives keep in touch with the firm's executive business."[1(p.1)]

The process is often referred to as 'walking the floor'. Here rather than administration from the executive suite, those in leadership or supervisory positions are regular participants 'where the action is'.

There appears to be an increasing tendency for occupational therapists in administrative or managerial positions to isolate themselves from the centre of the action, possibly seeking status from the trappings of the position. Concentrating on the management role and attending meetings, they are likely to manage in a vacuum and at the same time send another powerful negative message to front line service providers. Given the present findings about the values of occupational therapists, we should be able to design a management system within each unit to enable therapists to do what they value most highly—providing service to clients/patients with as much autonomy as possible. Care must be taken to match the degree of responsibility with the level of authority.

6. *"Stick to the knitting*—remaining with the business the company knows best."[1(p.1)]

Successful companies were those that stayed reasonably close to the business they knew. We shall refrain from giving attribute #6 any concrete interpretation, but this element appears to be the one that gives the occupational therapy profession its major stumbling block. What do occupational therapists do? What is the profession's specific contribution? What theoretical knowledge base is its foundation? How effective are the intervention procedures? Our search for professional identity spans decades and occurs in the occupational therapy literature of almost every English speaking country.

A variety of explanations have been offered, but there often appears to be little agreement. To reach such an agreement, collaborative research endeavours must become a reality. As long as the problem remains at the clinical level and the major source of expertise with which to investigate it is isolated within a university, progress is unlikely. As long as graduate programs in occupational therapy are in short supply, the best innovative thinkers will be lured to allied fields; therefore, the development of graduate programs must receive priority.

7. *"Simple form, lean staff*—few administrative layers, few people at the upper levels.''[1(p.1)]

Lean and simple are the key words here. Although there is nothing simple about a health care facility's organizational structure, economic reality alone will streamline middle management. Therefore, occupational therapy managers must be proactive. They must have accurate case load and cost data. They must know what type of service requests are most frequently received and the cost involved in meeting those demands. They must be prepared to identify areas of endeavour which can be dropped. Supervisors must become good negotiators to maintain the unit's identity and level of productivity.

8. *"Simultaneous loose-tight properties*—fostering a climate where there is dedication to the central values of the company combined with tolerance for all employees who accept these values.''[1(p.1)]

The question of centralization or decentralization is at issue here. Autonomy may be pushed down to the front line service team but the essential values, the core, are rigidly under central control.

There would appear to be some reluctance in the occupational therapy profession to allow creative, innovative therapists space to exercise their talents. It is almost as if there is no realization that the unit as a whole will benefit from their endeavors, not just the individuals themselves.

After isolating the unit's goals and deciding upon the objectives for the year or the quarter, the staff must then be free to get on with meeting those objectives. Managers must be ready to reward their staff's successful attainment. Find out what extrinsic elements within the job are most highly valued and allocate them when and where performance warrants.

CONCLUSION

Peters and Waterman stated that:

> The excellent companies seem to have developed cultures that have incorporated the values and the practices of the great leaders and thus those shared values can be seen to survive for decades . . . the real role of the chief executive officer is to manage the *values* of the organization.[1(p.26)]

Occupational therapy in Canada has a long and prestigious history, professional values have been established and great leaders have made contributions to professional development. Although the importance of the leader has been stressed throughout this discussion, hands-on managerial style, the role model, perhaps even the heroic stance, one individual is not enough " . . . it is the team at the top that is crucial".[1(p.290)] That is the real message.

Occupational therapy management is now being called upon to break some old habits and shift attention at the same time that our university programs are being required to adjust to similar pressures. The economic downturn can have some positive effects if department heads are willing to take a proactive stance, to open negotiations with well supported arguments. They must demonstrate that they are very much aware of the bottom line, and use all the resources inside and outside the clinical settings to bring the best brains together. Such a team will be able to devise the best solution to a problem and to demonstrate our professional effectiveness through action.

REFERENCES

1. Peters, TJ & Waterman, RH: In Search of Excellence. New York: Warner. 1983
2. Madill, HM: A Cross Sectional Analysis of Work Related Issues in Occupational Therapy. Unpublished doctoral dissertation, The University of Alberta, Edmonton, Alberta, Canada. 1985
3. Fitzsimmons, GW, Macnab, D & Casserly, MC: Life Roles Inventory Canadian National Norming Study 1984. Ottawa: Employment & Immigration Canada. 1984

4. Fitzsimmons, GW, Macnab, D & Casserly, MC: Life Roles Inventory Technical Manual. Ottawa: Employment & Immigration Canada. 1984

5. Casserly, MC: The identification of the importance of work. In NATCON I (Employment & Immigration Canada, pp. 121–129). Ottawa, Canada: Minister of Supply & Services Canada. 1982

6. Macnab, D: Work Related Needs, Preferences and Values: An Empirical Integration. Unpublished doctoral dissertation, The University of Alberta, Edmonton, Alberta, Canada. 1985

7. Goldenberg, K & Quinn, B: Community occupational therapy associates: A model of private practice for community occupational therapy. *Occupational Therapy in Health Care*, 2:15–22. 1985

Managing Occupational Therapy Burnout

Chestina Brollier, PhD, OTR, FAOTA
Jill Cyranowski, MS, OTR
Doreen Bender, MS, OTR
Carolyn Velletri, MS, OTR

ABSTRACT. Burnout has been conceptualized as an ineffective coping response to stress experienced on the job. This article will explore the construct of burnout as reported in the literature of the helping professions. An emphasis will be placed on prevention and remediation strategies, particularly those aimed at organizational causes of burnout for occupational therapists.

Burnout is an old phenomenon. Stress-related problems have been found to permeate the lives of many helping professionals. Nurses, physicians, social workers, physical therapists, and psychologists have all been found to experience problems identified as professional burnout.[2-4] Although occupational therapists have only recently been studied, the available data suggests that some occupational therapists employed in the United States may also have problems with burnout.[5,6]

CONCEPTS

Burnout has been conceptualized in the formal literature within the United States in several ways. Perlman and Hartman[7] based

Chestina Brollier is Assistant Professor, Occupational Therapy Department, Virginia Commonwealth University, Richmond, VA. Jill Cyranowski is a staff occupational therapist, Cumberland Hospital, New Kent, VA. Doreen Bender resides in Richmond, VA. Carolyn Velletri is a staff occupational therapist, Johnston-Willis Hospital, Richmond, VA.

This article appears jointly in *Occupational Therapy for People With Eating Dysfunctions* (The Haworth Press, Inc., 1986) and *Occupational Therapy in Health Care*, Volume 3, Number 2 (Summer 1986).

130   *Occupational Therapy for People With Eating Dysfunctions*

their definition on a content analysis of the burnout literature from 1974 to 1980. They defined burnout as a response to chronic emotional stress with three components: emotional or physical exhaustion, lowered job productivity, and depersonalization or lack of concern for others. Watkins,[8] after evaluating a number of definitions, cited the following three distinct identifying characteristics of burnout: depletion of physical and mental resources; personal expectations aimed too high; and relationships with others (e.g., patients) that sap one's reserves.

Whereas there are differences among these definitions, there are some common threads. Maslach[2] stated that there is general agreement that burnout occurs at an individual level; that burnout is an internal psychological experience involving feelings, attitudes, motives, and expectations; and that burnout is a negative experience for the individual. The following description by Maslach and Jackson[9] appears to be a widely accepted one. "Burnout is a syndrome of emotional exhaustion and cynicism that occurs frequently among individuals who do 'people work' ".[p.1]

SIGNS

Burnout is frequently described by the presence of symptoms rather than given a precise definition. There are a number of signs manifested in the burnout syndrome which Patrick[10] has categorized into four areas; behavioral, emotional, cognitive, and physical. Because of the large number and types of signs, Emener[1] emphasized that there mere existence is not the crucial element in the identification of burnout but rather that the frequency and magnitude of these indicators are the crucial elements.

Behaviorally, Freudenberger[12] observed that he did less work and worked less efficiently while experiencing burnout. A resistance to change[13] and a decrease in flexibility[4,10,12] are other behavioral indicators of the presence of burnout. A worker may begin to draw boundaries between the job and outside interests, known as compartmentalization.[4] Various types of withdrawal, including absenteeism[8,13] and withdrawal from personal and social life,[10,13] are other behavioral symptoms.

The emotional symptoms have been a focus of Maslach's and her colleagues' work.[2,3,9] While others[8,10,12] have noted general emotional changes, such as depression and helplessness, there has been considerable attention given to more specific emotional indicators of burnout. First, *emotional exhaustion* is considered to be a major sign of burnout.[4,9,10] A negative shift in attitudes toward patients and a lack of concern for those with whom one works, termed *depersonalization*, is another emotional sign of burnout.[2-4,9,10,13] Finally, a decrease in the worker's self-image may reflect burnout.[2,3,9,10] Maslach and Jackson[2] have expanded the concept and termed it *reduced personal accomplishment*.

In addition to behavioral and emotional signs, there are cognitive and physical signs of burnout. Cognitive indicators, the third category outlined by Patrick,[10] include a decreased ability to solve problems and make decisions and a general alteration of the individual's typical cognitive style.[8] Physically, an individual may manifest fatigue or extreme physical exhaustion,[2-4,8-10,12,13] sleep and eating disturbances,[10] and psychosomatic symptoms.[14]

CONSEQUENCES

The many consequences of burnout affect the individual, his or her patients, the organization, and reach out of the work environment into virtually all aspects of the individual's life. The professional may suffer emotional and physical exhaustion, a diminished self-concept, and alcohol or drug abuse. Performance on the job may be impaired.[13-15] The consequences to the patient include dehumanization[16] and a decreased quality of services.[17] Poor staff morale,[14,17] increased absenteeism, higher staff turnover and a decrease in average length of stay on the job[14] are very serious consequences of burnout to the organization. Although burnout originates from work-related stress, its consequences are also felt in marriages and families.[4,13,14]

To increase our understanding of burnout, a number of causal factors have been identified. These causes will be examined now.

CAUSES OF BURNOUT

The burnout syndrome is believed to result from chronic occupational stress. In reviewing occupational sources of stress, Cooper and Marshall[18] have suggested three central sources of stress: individual characteristics of the person, potential sources of stress in the work environment, and extra-organizational sources of stress such as family problems, financial difficulties, and life crises.

Individual causes. Personal causes of burnout may include the following characteristics of the person: personality, locus of control, coping styles, extreme idealism, and others. Freudenberger[12] suggested several personality types that are prone to burnout. These include the dedicated and committed worker, the overcommitted worker whose nonwork life is subsatisfactory, and the authoritarian personality. Helliwell[19] described the susceptible individual as one who is idealistic and who has a single-minded purpose for his or her life.

Locus of control,[20] the degree to which an individual perceives that he or she has personal control over outcomes, has been suggested as another characteristic that may cause burnout.[21] Maslach[22] indicated that both undercontrol and overcontrol in helping situations contribute to burnout.

A number of other characteristics of the individual may lead to burnout. Because it results from chronic occupational stress, an individual's coping style will influence susceptiblity or resistance to the burnout syndrome.[21] Individuals who begin their jobs at the extreme of idealistic over-involvement may be particularly vulnerable to burnout.[11,12,21]

Organizational causes. The largest portion of literature has focused upon characteristics of the work environment that cause burnout. Maslach[22] concluded that burnout is best understood in terms of the social and situational sources of job-related stresses. Organizational causes involve the relationships between the worker and the organization, the patients, and co-workers.

There are a number of potential causes of burnout resulting from the worker-organization relationship. Many aspects of the work environment, such as policy and decision-making, may be beyond a worker's authority resulting in a lack of control and feelings of helplessness.[2,21] With opportunities for control lacking in the environment, the worker feels trapped and may be more prone to burnout.

Role ambiguity and role conflict have been identified as sources of stress within the worker-organization relationship. Role ambiguity occurs when the worker lacks the relevant information necessary for adequate performance of the job. Two types of information identified as particularly important in determining stress reactions are information about the job tasks to be performed and information about how others evaluate the worker.[2] Role conflict results from the incompatability of demands, and it may be in the form of conflict between organizational demands and one's own values, problems of personal resource allocation, conflict between obligations to several other people, or conflict between excessively numerous or difficult tasks.[23] Role conflict and ambiguity have been correlated with burnout in child care workers[24] and have been suggested as a cause of burnout in other health-related professions.[3,4] Closely related to role ambiguity and conflict is the lack of recognition of one's work. Inadequate feedback is thought to be a causal factor in burnout.[3,10,21]

A heavy workload is another antecedent to burnout.[4,10,13,24] Particularly in health-related professions where the worker is expected to adequately care for many patients, too much to do in too little time may lead to stress. The fact that health professionals are responsible for people rather than things[25] adds to the perceived stress. Furthermore, these patients are people with problems.

Another cause of burnout in the worker-organization relationship is lack of perceived success. Health professionals, including occupational therapists, expect to help their patients and preferably to cure them. In reality, the patients who require most of the attention and time of occupational therapists are often severely and chronically disabled. Because there are no cures[11,26] and because patients often expect "cures" from health professionals, they both will be disappointed. According to Wolfe,[4] a primary antecedent to burnout in physical therapists appears to be an inability on the part of the therapist to perceive success in the treatment of patients, particularly in the rehabilitation or maintenance of the chronically ill patient.

Finally, the work milieu may be a predisposing factor in burnout.[10,25] A work setting can be nurturing or barren. Patrick[10] has suggested that chronic exposure to an environment that lacks stimulation or variation can elicit apathy toward the setting, dissatisfaction with work produced within the setting, or lack of desire to enter the setting.

One organizational cause of burnout now receiving a great deal of attention, particularly in the health professions, is the therapist-patient relationship. Sources of burnout in the therapist-patient relationship include the amount of contact with patients,[3,21,22] the type and severity of the patient's problem[3,22] and the interactions between therapist and patient,[3,21,22] among others. The amount of contact with patients is an important factor in burnout because of the emotional aspects of the helping relationship. The more time spent in direct care, the greater the risk of the emotional exhaustion component of burnout.[3] Also, the staff-patient ratio was found to be related to greater job stress for workers in mental health facilities.[27]

Similarly, the type of patient's problem is another potential source of stress. In health professions, workers may be involved with patients who have severe and debilitating disabilities. Once again, the chronicity of the condition is a factor. For example, staff members who worked with a high percentage of schizophrenics in the patient population expressed less job satisfaction in one study.[27]

A number of things can affect therapist-patient interactions and therefore their relationship. Maslach[22] discussed a number of explicit and implicit rules, another source of stress, that structure the interaction between a therapist and patient. For example, explicit rules may limit the amount of time a staff member can devote to a patient and implicit rules may require a passive, dependent patient. The quantity and quality of communication and the amount and type of feedback may also affect the relationship. Pines and Maslach[27] found that the quality of interaction between mental health workers and their patients was positively related to the worker's perceptions of the institution, of other staff members, of the work, and of the patients. The nature of the therapist-patient relationship is an important consideration in the burnout syndrome of a health professional.

Another organizational variable thought to mediate burnout is the availability and use of social supports and feedback from fellow workers.[21] Relationships with co-workers, including the supervisor, colleagues, and team members have been cited as a factor in burnout among social workers.[25] When supportive co-workers are available, burnout is less prevalent.[28]

Administrators are also prone to these same organizational stressors. Although managers might spend less time with patients, the administrator-staff relationship is similar to the one between staff and patients.[29] Moreover, there are stressors specifically identified with the administrative role. Harvey and Raider[29] discussed the following administrative stressors: relationships with funding bodies, inter-organizational relationships, accountability to consumers and funding sources, and being a ''linchpin'' between the needs and perceptions of the staff and the demands and constraints of the external environment. Furthermore, Harvey and Raider[29] related that if "the administrator has been trained as a direct service professional rather than a manager, the potential for conflict and stress may be magnified" (p.84). Therefore, managers may be prone to burnout because of additional organizational stressors.

In summary, organizational causes of stress in the work environment include relationships between the worker and the organization, the patients, and co-workers. Managers are subject to experiencing the same stressors as their staff in addition to ones specific to their administrative roles.

Environmental causes. In addition to individual and organizational causes of burnout, extra-organizational sources of stress may contribute to the burnout syndrome. Doohan[30] discussed several characteristics of the time in which we live. The sheer weight of change and our society's narrow perception of leisure, for example, may contribute to burnout. Cherniss[31] has suggested that other aspects of society contribute to burnout in human service occupations. The recently instituted Prospective Payment System for Medicare, often termed DRGs, and the resultant push for productivity is an aspect affecting many health professionals such as occupational therapists. Stresses in one's personal life[10] may also affect how one deals with stress on the job.

Individual characteristics of a worker and sources of stress outside of the workplace are important. However, the largest portion of literature and empirical research has revolved around the organizational causes of burnout.

STAGES

Burnout does not "develop overnight". Freudenberger[12] referred to the development of burnout in dedicated and committed workers. Initially, individuals worked harder and longer to accomplish tasks. Eventually, they became frustrated and exhausted in their attempts to complete their work. Cynicism or apathy was often the end result. Others who have addressed the stages of burnout[26,30] have discussed a similar development of the burnout syndrome. However, stages of burnout, in general, do not comprise a major part of the burnout literature.

PREVENTION AND REMEDIATION OF BURNOUT

Burnout is a serious personal and occupational dysfunction. Preventive and coping techniques for burnout can be categorized as either personal or organizational strategies. According to Patrick,[10] the goals of a burnout care program should include prevention, intervention, and management. When burnout develops in an organization, it is highly contagious.[31,32] Also, when one staff member burns out, reversing the condition often requires an extended effort. Therefore, prevention should be emphasized. Most occupational therapists seem to be familiar with the personal prevention strategies that follow, and many therapists may use the organizational strategies that are presented. This report simply tries to describe the scope of methods available.

Personal Prevention and Remediation

Personal prevention and coping strategies consist of the general life style of the individual and techniques over which he or she has control. Preventive strategies include a well-balanced life style in the areas of work, rest, and leisure. One area, for example, work, should not be overindulged in and another area such as leisure excluded. Doohan[30] has emphasized the need for proper nutrition, regular exercise, and time for leisure in the prevention of burnout. Interaction with well-adjusted healthy individuals when one works with a disabled population is another measure.[8] Pines and Maslach[27] have encouraged the individual to be aware of work stresses, to set realistic professional and personal goals, to meet one's own needs (in addition to the patients'), and to recognize the signs of burnout. A "decompression routine"[3,22] between leaving work and home, such as physical exercise, is a measure that may also prevent strain in the home environment.

Other personal ways of coping include relaxation or stress reduction techniques such as yoga and progressive muscle relaxation.[4,10,12,21] Although there are numerous techniques to prevent and to cope with burnout on an individual basis, they may be overlooked or ignored. Burnout is associated with chronic stress on the job. Therefore, individuals may focus on the job as the problem and not consider individual coping mechanisms outside the work environment. In many cases they may not even perceive themselves as suffering from burnout. A major step toward prevention and remediation is recognition of symptoms within oneself. A number of organizational strategies for dealing with burnout also exist.

Organizational Prevention and Remediation

There are five major points of organizational intervention: staff development, job and role structure, management development, organizational problem-solving, and program goals and philosophies.[31] Although they overlap, each of these will be separately discussed. Of course, the use of any intervention should be based on an analysis of the problems experienced by the staff and managers in the particular setting. As the interventions are used, their effectiveness, as well as unintended consequences, should be assessed.

Staff Development

Even modest staff development interventions have been reported to reduce burnout.[31,32] For example, Weitz[33] has reported on the effectiveness of using an orientation booklet that described typical examples of the kinds of frustrations and disappointments one might encounter on the job. Although novice occupational therapists have received considerable training and fieldwork, a thorough, realistic orientation program can communicate that they are not expected to be fully competent from the beginning. This can reduce excessively ambitious goals, which have been found to be a precursor to burnout in often idealistic new professionals.

Another staff development method is the "burnout checkup".[31] Approximately twice a year, each staff member meets with a staff development specialist to discuss current sources of stress and satisfaction experienced on the job. The specialist must be someone other than the direct supervisor. The findings from this assessment are used to help each staff member and the department make changes in jobs. This evaluation can also be used as a basis for further individual consultation and group or departmental interventions.[34] Resource networks and support groups that allow professionals to share experiences and adaptive mechanisms also reportedly reduce burnout. These networks help professionals realize that their stressors are not unique to them and that there are adequate adaptive mechanisms available.[32] In summary, staff development methods can assist occupational therapists in alleviating negative consequences of some job stressors.

Job Structure

Although staff development can often reduce burnout, it frequently must be combined with alterations in jobs to have major benefits in reducing stress. The two basic sources of job stress are (1) external demands that exceed the individual's resources and (2) lack of opportunity to do the type of work one finds most rewarding.[31] Jobs can be altered to reduce work overload, conflict, and ambiguity. Enriching jobs through increasing opportunities for stimulation, variety, and learning should also be a goal.[31,32] Individual preferences of staff must be considered.

Even though occupational therapy managers must be concerned with the productivity of staff, each staff member should be assigned only a reasonable number of patients and the most difficult, unrewarding work should, of course, be distributed fairly among staff. Staff can be helped to arrange their schedules so that rewarding and unrewarding activities are alternated to some extent. For example, paper work and other time away from patients can be interspersed with patient treatment. Volunteers and para-professionals need to be used when appropriate. Staff members should not be expected to routinely take work home or spend excessive hours on the job. Use of part-time staff and flexible work hours for staff should also be considered.

Another recommendation is that staff members be encouraged to design and implement new treatment programs. This process can further commitment and satisfaction even in demanding jobs.[31] One last recommendation for alleviating burnout through job structure is to develop realistic career ladders for staff. Significant increases in responsibility, privileges, and rewards for competent work can increase satisfaction with work.[31]

Management Development

"Research has suggested that differences in the quality of supervision and leadership account for more of the variance in burnout than any other single factor".[31,p.176] Managers, whether or not they realize their power, do influence their staff member's stressors. Also, in one study of hospital-based occupational therapy managers, the managers reported more intense feelings of depersonalization and emotional exhuastion than staff OTRs.[5] Thus, at least one sample of occupational therapy managers were experiencing burnout that appeared to be related to their managerial duties.

Poor supervision and management are usually caused by either naive attitudes, lack of skill, and/or excessive role demands on the manager.[31] Management development may need to address all three of these areas.

One suggestion to decrease burnout in occupational therapy managers and ultimately in their staff is to improve the managerial training and skills of occupational therapists. This might be achieved by any of the following. A post-professional master's degree in occupational therapy management should be developed in universities across the United States. Another idea proposed by Shuff[35] is to offer an optional administrative fieldwork II to professional master's degree candidates. Realistically, these students often accept management positions early in their careers, and the optional fieldwork may more adequately prepare them for the jobs. Management continuing education workshops need to be available on at least a regional basis. While these could not take the place of advanced education, they would be useful to administrators who are unable to return to school. Management consulting services would also be helpful in quickly identifying problems in a department and steering the administrator toward effective solutions. This might reduce the stress that managers experience when they are unable to solve a problem and have no one to turn to for advice.

Managers who also provide patient treatment and thus are at risk for work overload may respond positively to approaches that structure their job more for them. Occupational therapy managers also may need regular feedback on their performance and someone to periodically assist in monitoring their role strain. Managers, just as staff, could profit from burnout ''check-ups''.

Managers may need specialized training in what has been called creative supervision.[32] This approach seems to be particularly useful with staff who are experiencing low feelings of personal accomplishment.[2] Creative supervision is characterized by a high degree of support from the supervisor, which does not reduce the worker's autonomy. Supervision should help the OTR enhance technical skills, thus helping the OTR feel more competent; and promote self-esteem, thus increasing feelings of success. Maintaining clear communication channels between supervisor and employee is also important in making supervision a successful process.

Well trained occupational therapy managers can assist staff OTRs in dealing with the bureaucracy encountered in many facilities. Managers can support their staff by acting as buffers and advocates between the worker and the organization. Workers often feel powerless against bureaucracies. If they know that their occupational therapy manager is supporting their interests when dealing with higher administration, they may feel more in control and burnout may be reduced.[31] Brollier[36] has found that when managers exhibited skills in being a strong leader, able to negotiate effectively with superiors, staff job satisfaction was high.

Occupational therapy managers whose departments are affected by the Medicare Prospective Payment System may particularly need specialized training. In one study, the levels of burnout for OTRs working in occupational therapy departments affected by the DRGs were higher than those OTRs whose departments were not included under DRGs.[5] As well as allowing staff to have increased job control, managers dealing with DRGs can reduce stress and increase productivity by developing streamlined record keeping, offering flex-time so employees can work the hours when they are most productive and when they are needed, and specializing in disabilities that the department treats most successfully. Instructing staff on time management techniques and encouraging them to keep their own productivity statistics may further increase departmental productivity.[31] Garibaldi[37] has noted that more occupational therapy service is being demanded in a shorter time period, and that patients are being discharged earlier with the onset of the DRGs. Effective management skills are vital to successfully implement these changes in occupational therapy departments.

Organizational Problem-Solving

Even the best managed programs experience conflicts. When problems are examined in a crisis atmosphere, today's solutions often become tomorrow's problems.[31] Consequently, another area of burnout intervention must be problem-solving and conflict resolution.

Formal mechanisms must be developed for departmental problem-solving. First, occupational therapy managers need to learn to use a variety of conflict resolution methods and to be able to match the methods to the problems presented. One study of a large sample of hospital-based occupational therapists found that the occupational therapy manager's conflict resolution abilities correlated rather highly with staff job satisfaction and to a lesser extent with staff job performance.[36,38] Thus, management training for occupational therapists should include conflict resolution. Practical books on the subject can also be useful to staff as well as managers.

Another recommendation is that participative decision-making be appropriately used. The management literature and research has produced guidelines for this.[39] When staff members have particular expertise and interest in a subject, when they will be directly influenced by the decisions, and when there is adequate time for group problem-solving, then staff should be most involved. Participative management is successful when professional staff members are also given adequate autonomy and control over their jobs.[39] Some common reasons why managers fail to delegate routine matters to their staff include a lack of experience in how to delegate authority, a lack of confidence in subordinates, and a fear that subordinates will not like them if they delegate work.[39] Participatory management has been found to be related to increased job satisfaction when staff are consulted about issues that not only interest them, but also on issues that they are competent to address.[39]

Philosophies and Goals

Burnout appears to be less severe when there is a strong sense of shared purpose in a department.[31,32] The development of a distinctive guiding philosophy of treatment can be an effective mechanism for synthesizing a program's focus. Thus, occupational therapy managers and staff may want to examine the underlying values and principles upon which they base their programming. From this process a series of goals for the program can be produced. Clear, consistent work goals have been linked to job satisfaction and reduced burnout.[39]

SUMMARY AND CONCLUSIONS

Burnout is a response to stress experienced on the job. Job stress occurs when there is an imbalance between job demands and an individual's skills, time, and energy.[31] The person's preferences and goals also create demands that can produce stress. Occupational therapists and many other helping professionals seem to be at risk for burnout. There exist as many ways of dealing with burnout as causes. Personal strategies have only briefly been reviewed here. Organizational methods of prevention and remediation of burnout in the work environment were emphasized in the review for two reasons. First, differences in jobs and organizations probably are more powerful sources of burnout than are differences in the individual.[30] Secondly, it is ultimately easier to reduce the incidence and severity of burnout by intervening at the organizational level.[30] Interventions at the organizational level not only tend to be more effective, but they also have potential for affecting more individuals with the same resources.[30] The strategies presented here will ultimately be effective for occupational therapists only if they are matched to specific situations, carefully monitored, and not imposed upon individuals.

REFERENCES

1. Richardson M, West P: Motivational management: Coping with burnout. *Hosp & Community Psychiatry* 33: 837–840, 1982

2. Maslach C: Burnout: The High Cost of Caring, Englewood Cliffs, NJ: Prentice Hall, 1982

3. Maslach C, Jackson S: Burnout in health professions: A social psychological analysis. In Social Psychology of Health and Illness, G Sanders, J Suls, Editors. Hillsdale, NJ: Lawrence Erlbaum, Assoc, 1982

4. Wolfe G: Burnout of therapists: Inevitable or preventable. *Physical Therapy* 61: 1046–1050, 1981

5. Brollier C, Bender D, Cyranowski J, Velletri C: A pilot study of job burnout in hospital-based occupational therapists. *Occup Ther J of Research* (in press)

6. Brollier C, Velletri C, Cyranowski J, Bender D: A comparison of OTR burnout to Maslach Burnout Inventory norms. *Am J Occup Ther* (in press)

7. Perlman B, Hartman E: Burnout: Summary and future research. *Human Relations* 35: 283–305, 1982

8. Watkins C: Burnout in counseling practice; Some potential professional and personal hazards of becoming a counselor. *Personnel and Guidance J* 61: 304–308, 1983

9. Maslach C, Jackson S: Maslach Burnout Inventory, Palo Alto: Consulting Psychologists Press, Inc., 1981

10. Patrick P: Burnout: Job hazard for health workers. *Hospitals*, Nov 16; 87–90, 1979

11. Emener W: Professional burnout: Rehabilitation's hidden handicap. *J of Rehab*, Jan–March; 55–58, 1979

12. Freudenberger H: The staff burnout syndrome in alternative institutions. *Psychotherapy: Theory, Research and Practice*, 12: 73–82, 1975

13. Weiskopf P: Burnout among teachers of exceptional children. *Exceptional Children* 47: 18–23, 1980

14. Maslach C, Jackson S: Burnout-out cops and their families. *Psychology Today* 12; 59–62, 1979

15. Zabel R, Zabel M: Factors in burnout among teachers of exceptional children. *Exceptional Children* 49: 261–263, 1982

16. Maslach C, Pines A: The burn-out syndrome in the day care setting. *Child Care Quarterly*, 6: 100–113, 1977

17. Carroll J, White W: Theory building: Integrating individual and environmental factors within an ecological framework. In Job Stress and Burnout: Research, Theory, and Intervention Perspectives, W Paine, Editor. Beverly Hills: Sage, 1982

18. Cooper C, Marshall J: Occupational sources of stress: A review of the literature relating to coronary heart disease and mental ill health. *J Occup Psychology* 49: 11–28, 1976

19. Helliwell T: Are you a potential burnout? *Training and Development J* 35: 25–29, 1981

20. Rotter J: Generalized expectancies for internal versus external control of reinforcement. *Psych Monographs* 80, 1966

21. Savicki V, Cooley E: Implications of burnout research and theory for counselor educators. *Personnel and Guidance J* 60: 415–419, 1982

22. Maslach C: The client role in staff burn-out. *J of Social Issues* 34: 111–124, 1978

23. Cook J, Hepworth S, Wall T, Warr, P: The Experience of Work: A Compendium and Review of 249 Measures and Their Use, London: Academic Press, 1981

24. Jayaratne S, Chess W: Job satisfaction, burnout, and turnover: A national study. *Social Work* 29: 448–453, 1984

25. Taylor-Brown S, Johnson K, Hunter K, Rockowitz R: Stress identification for social workers in health care: A preventive approach to burnout. *Social Work in Health Care* 7: 91–100, 1981

26. Burnett-Beaulieu S: Occupational therapy profession dropouts: Escape from the grief process. *Occupational Therapy in Mental Health* 2: 45–55, 1982

27. Pines A, Maslach C: Characteristics of staff burnout in mental health settings. *Hosp and Community Psychiatry* 29: 233–237, 1978

28. Pines A, Kafry D: Occupational tedium in social service professionals. *Social Work* 23: 499–507, 1978

29. Harvey S, Raider M: Administrator burnout. *Administration in Social Work* 8: 81–89, 1984

30. Doohan H: Burnout: A critical issue for the 1980s. *J of Religion and Health* 21: 352–358, 1982

31. Cherniss C: Staff Burnout: Job Stress in The Human Services, Beverly Hills: Sage, 1980

32. Paine W: Job Stress and Burnout: Research, Theory, and Intervention perspectives, Beverly Hills: Sage, 1982

33. Weitz J: Job expectancy and survival. *J Applied Psych* 40: 245–247, 1956

34. Caplan G: The Theory and Practice of Mental Health Consultation, NY: Basic Books, 1970

35. Shuff F: The need for specific training in administration for professional growth. *Am J Occup Ther* 20: 28–30, 1966

36. Brollier C: Managerial leadership and staff OTR job satisfaction. *Occup Ther J of Research* 5: 170–184, 1985

37. Garibaldi J: Survey Findings: Impact of Medicare Prospective Payment System on Occupational Therapy, Rockville, MD: AOTA, 1985

38. Brollier C: A study of Occupational therapy management and job performance of staff. *Am J Occup Ther* (in press)

39. Yukl G: Leadership in Organizations, Englewood Cliffs, NJ: Prentice Hall, 1981

SOMETHING NEW AND USEFUL. . .

The RIC Combination Short-Opponens Pushcuff Orthosis

Elizabeth B. Mason, OTR/L
Kathleen A. Okkema, MBA, OTR/L

Occupational therapists are often faced with the dilemma of maintaining proper client hand position for activities while at the same time promoting function. For the person with spinal cord injury, the importance of maintaining the integrity of hand structures has been documented by many authors.[1-6] The combination short-opponens pushcuff orthosis was developed at the Rehabilitation Institute of Chicago (RIC) in order to promote proper hand position during wheelchair propulsion. The orthosis has been effective in preventing deformity caused by stretching of the thumb musculature. The functional tenodesis pinch necessary for performance of daily living skills is therefore preserved.

Elizabeth B. Mason is staff occupational therapist, Kathleen A. Okkema is Clinical Education Specialist in Occupational Therapy at R.I.C., which is part of Northwestern-McGaw Medical Center, Chicago, IL.

The authors would like to thank the Rehabilitation Institute of Chicago, Sharon Intigliata, MS, MPA, OTR/L; Patricia Conlon, MA, OTR/L and the Biomedical Media Services Department for their time and support; special thanks as well to those occupational therapists who helped design the pushcuff orthosis, particularly Jereen Mackefy, OTR/L.

This article appears jointly in *Occupational Therapy for People With Eating Dysfunctions* (The Haworth Press, Inc., 1986) and *Occupational Therapy in Health Care*, Volume 3, Number 2 (Summer 1986).

BACKGROUND

Wheelchair pushcuffs (Figure 1) are frequently issued to C 6-8 quadriplegic clients at RIC. Further, however, because the push-cuff is not a positioning device, use of this device alone was observed to cause stretching of the flexor and adductor muscles of the thumb. This stretching led to deterioration of functional tenodesis prehension. The RIC combination short-opponens push-cuff orthosis (Figures 2 and 3) was developed therefore to pro-vide proper thumb positioning during the day as well as safe wheelchair propulsion. The orthosis consists of a custom-made thermoplastic short-opponens splint riveted to a leather wheelchair pushcuff. The addition to the regular cuff of the short-opponens orthosis ensures proper thumb positioning essential to functional pinch and yet does not interfere with one's ability to hand propel a wheelchair.

ADVANTAGES

The combination pushcuff orthosis:

1. maintains natural tenodesis by stabilizing the thumb in opposition,
2. preserves or replaces pinch in those clients lacking thumb strength or position,
3. is easy to put on and take off,
4. is cost effective,
5. is easy to fabricate, requiring few materials.

CONSIDERATIONS FOR FABRICATION

1. Early fabrication and fitting of the pushcuff orthosis has been clinically shown to improve compliance with orthotic wear.
2. Because significant pressure must be applied to the hand during wheelchair propulsion, it is important that the thermo-plastic orthotic portion fit well.

3. If positioning the thumb in opposition is painful, the pushcuff orthosis would be contraindicated and other means of positioning should be explored.

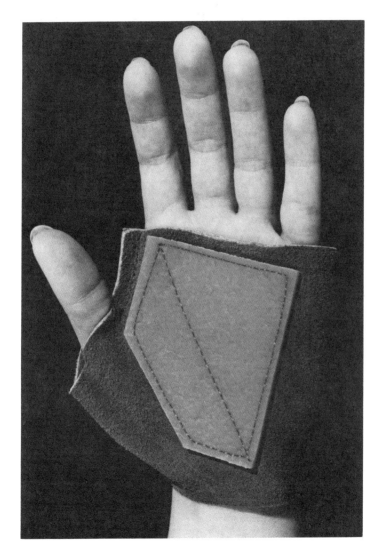

FIGURE 1. Example of commercially-available leather pushcuff.

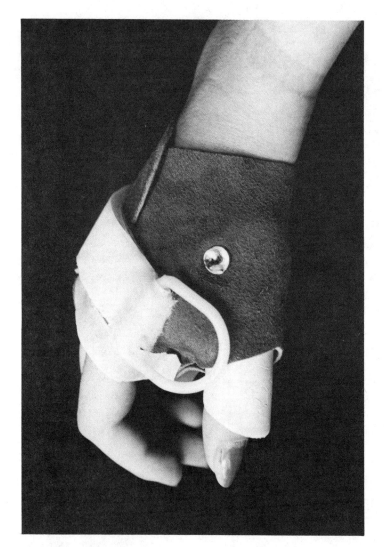

FIGURE 2. Short opponens-pushcuff orthosis with metal rivet and D-ring velcro closure.

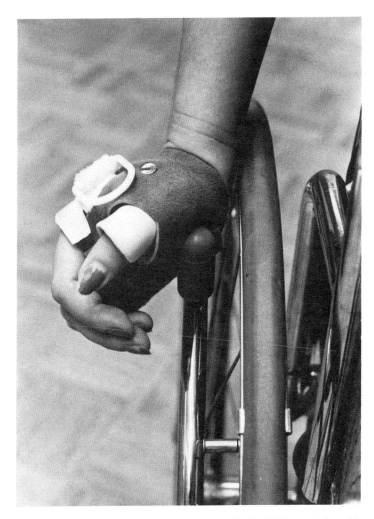

FIGURE 3. Short opponens-pushcuff orthosis used in wheelchair propulsion with a C$_6$ quadriplegic client.

Although the orthosis was orginally designed for quadriplegic clients, it has also proven functional for other wheelchair-bound clients with diagnoses such as peripheral neuropathy, multiple sclerosis and Guillain-Barré syndrome. The pushcuff adaptation is also currently being used successfully in conjunction with long-opponens orthoses and with lumbrical bar attachments (Figure 4).

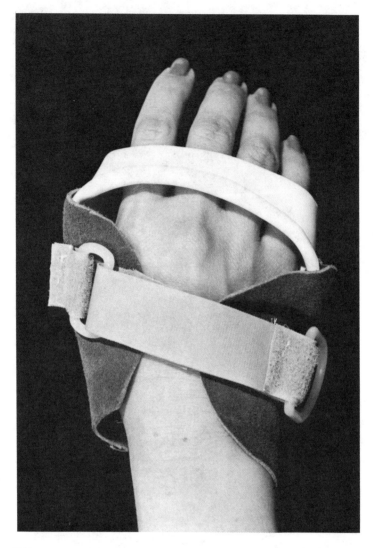

FIGURE 4. Overhead view of short-opponens pushcuff orthosis with lumbrical bar attachment.

While the combination short-opponens pushcuff orthosis has been in use at RIC for one year, the effects of long term wear will be investigated through research beginning within the Institute.

LIST OF REFERENCES

American Academy of Orthopaedic Surgeons: Atlas of Orthotics. St. Louis: The C.V. Mosby Co., 1975, pp 63, 106, 118

Crenshaw A H, Edmonson A S: Campbell's Operative orthopaedics, Vol. I. St. Louis: the C.V. Mosby Co., 1980, pp. 275, 276

Di Pasquale P A: "The Use of Positioning Orthotics for Development of a Functional C_6 Quadriplegic Hand." Unpublished Manuscript, 1985

Hunter, Schneider, Mackin, Callihan: Rehabilitation Of The Hand. St. Louis: The C.V. Mosby Co., 1984, p 452

Malick, M H, Meyer, C M H: Manual on Management of the Quadriplegic Upper Extremity. Pittsburgh, 1978, pp 34–38

Trombly, C A: Occupational Therapy for Physical Dysfunction, Second Edition. Baltimore: Williams and Wilkins, 1983, p 265

BOOK REVIEWS

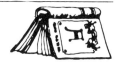

OCCUPATIONAL THERAPY PRACTICE SKILLS FOR PHYS-
ICAL DYSFUNCTION (2nd Ed.). Lorraine Williams Pedretti, MS,
OTR. *The C. V. Mosby Company, P.O. Box 28430, St. Louis, MO
63416. 1985, 477 pp, $34.95*

This book is designed for use by occupational therapy students in
baccalaureate and entry level master's degree programs in preparation for treatment of adults with acquired physical disabilities. The
topics covered are essentially the same as in *Occupational Therapy
for Physical Dysfunction*, (2nd edition), edited by Catherine Anne
Trombly, OTR. The organization and emphasis, however, are
slightly different. Explicit instruction on basic evaluation procedures, treatment methods, techniques, treatment objectives and
planning are emphasized more in this book. There is slightly more
background information given on a variety of dysfunctions and
disabilities which is necessary before beginning occupational therapy evaluation and treatment. The scope of occupational therapy
treatment methods and techniques is not quite as broad in this book
and there is not the emphasis on research to assist with conclusions
about effectiveness of specific treatment.

There are several unique features which lend this book well for
use in the academic setting. It is clearly organized according to the
occupational therapy process into sections on Foundations for
Treatment of Physical Dysfunction, Evaluation of Patients with
Physical Dysfunction, Treatment Methods, and Treatment Applications for patients with specific disabilities. Each chapter concludes
with review questions designed to aid in learning the material. At
the end of each chapter on treatment application a case study and
sample occupational therapy treatment plan are presented.

153

In this edition there are seven new chapters as well as several changes and additions to each remaining chapter. The direction of change was toward more detailed background information, i.e., medical considerations, description of dysfunction, neurological and physiological basis for treatment, more detailed instructions for specific procedures, and inclusion of lower extremity information and current advances in knowledge and techniques. Several additional authors contributed to this edition. Also, the format was changed to include more information on each page with smaller pictures and print.

Some of the explicit instructions are difficult to follow and additional pictures which might help with clarity were not used, i.e., the gravity eliminated positions on the manual muscle test, and the upper extremity prosthetic checkout procedure. Some of the sample forms appear "dated" by the language used. The current orthotic terminology is not consistently used. These are the major weaknesses noted.

Highlights of this edition are many. The first chapter presents occupational performance as a frame of reference for occupational therapy in physical dysfunction. It is an excellent introduction because it describes how the different methods and approaches to treatment fit together into this holistic frame of reference. One of the new chapters in the evaluation section is on muscle tone and coordination. It is typical of the chapters in this section as it presents useful background information, defines terms, presents purposes, methods, sample forms and treatment planning ideas as well as suggestions for assessment. The driving evaluation is an addition to the chapter on evaluation of performance skills. The chapters on sensorimotor approaches to treatment are particularly well done. The new chapter on neurophysiology of sensorimotor approaches presents a basis for treatment which includes conclusions from research supporting their use. The Rood and the Bobath approaches were expanded and the proprioceptive neuromuscular facilitation approach was added. The theoretical foundations as well as treatment techniques are outlined in enough detail to use them in treatment. The chapters on therapeutic activities and activities of daily living give specific treatment suggestions with helpful charts and pictures including an addition on quadriplegia dressing techniques. The chapter on wheelchairs and wheelchair transfers gives specific information for patient management as well as wheelchair ordering. The hand splinting information is geared toward critical theoretical aspects, i.e., normal hand function and principles of splinting with little on specific orthoses. The chapter including mobile arm supports is short and basic but a good introduction to a complicated subject. Cardiac dysfunction, low back pain, and hip fractures and total hip replacement were added to the section on treatment application. These follow the same format as the other chapters in this section on amputations, burns, rheumatoid arthritis, acute hand injuries, lower motor neuron dysfunction, spinal cord injury, cerebral vascular accident and head injury in adults. They each present background information necessary for occupational therapy evaluation and treatment as well as key points on basic assessment, treatment planning methods, ending with a case study and sample occupational therapy treatment plan.

It appears to this reviewer that this book succeeds in the mission for which it was designed. It is well suited for use with occupational therapy students in an academic setting where discussion and demonstration can supplement the basic well presented material on occupation therapy for adults with physical dysfunction.

Edith Gillespie, MEd, OTR

SPINAL CORD INJURY. Dorothy J. Wilson, BS, OTR, FAOTA, Mary W. McKenzie, MA, OTR, FAOTA, Lois M. Barber, BS. *Slack, Inc., 6900 Grove Rd., Thorofare, NJ 08086. 1984, $12.00.*

Spinal Cord Injury is an updated edition of the 1974 SCI treatment guide for occupational therapists from Rancho Los Amigos Hospital (RLAH). It follows the previous format. Graphic photographs and line drawings (some new, some old) are excellent.

Some of the new information included is on upper extremity tendon transfer surgeries and related sensory test changes, wheelchair and bed positioning, progressive casting, edema control, body handling skills, home and community skills and ADL, with more emphasis on a problem solving approach. New information on the Rachet Wrist Hand Orthosis has replaced that on the Electrically Powered Flexor Hinge Orthosis for C5 patients.

Although much orthotic terminology is updated in this edition, most of the orthotic information, especially that on mobile arm supports, is the thorough classic information RLAH has made available for many years. New material is offered on respiratory functioning and (for higher level quadriplegics) mouthstick options are presented. Other rapidly changing technology important to the C4 and above population, such as electric recline wheelchair options and environmental control units, is not included.

More driving options for quadriplegics are noted and a current catalogue of audio-visual aids on various aspects of SCI, from RLAH, is available.

This book is an excellent reference for any occupational therapist treating SCI patients. It provides guidelines for functional expectations at each level with most of the equipment needed, and information on how to attain these goals and utilize the equipment.

Juanita Ainsley, OTR

FUNCTIONAL ASSESSMENT IN REHABILITATION MEDICINE. Carl V. Granger, MD and Glen E. Gresham, MD, Editors. *Williams and Wilkins, 428 E. Preston St., Baltimore, MD 21202. 1984, 407pp, $42.00.*

Functional Assessment in Rehabilitation Medicine presents an interesting discussion of the need for indepth functional evaluation following illness or injury. The editors and contributors, who are largely physicians, begin by presenting an organized review of standard terminology and classification of disablement, and then build on this in succeeding chapters to validate the need for functional assessments. Currently available instruments are presented along with some research applications. Case examples from the aged, arthritic, amputee and mentally retarded populations are used to demonstrate how functional assessments may be applied. Quality of care and the need for benefit-cost analysis are also explored.

This would be an excellent textbook for use by educators, and as a resource for clinical administrators or therapists interested in research, to assist in documenting the effectivness of treatment. Although regrettably the authors very rarely mention occupational therapy, their subject and direction is the core of occupational therapy practice. The main goal of the authors appears to be pointing to the need for functional assessments as bases for determining treatment effectiveness, to justify payment for services, and to confirm the use of various treatment techniques. Students of research in occupational therapy would benefit from the information in the book as a guide and motivator in choosing thesis topics that would justify the need for or the effectiveness of treatment in objective ways. For the practicing occupational therapist, the book would encourage continuing in the direction in which the profession has already been moving—validating improvements in patient function by using careful assessment.

Karen Paris, OTR

AGING AND DEVELOPMENTAL DISABILITIES, ISSUES AND APPROACHES. Edited by Matthew P. Janicki, and Henry M. Wisniewski, Foreword by Gunnar Dybwad. *Paul H. Brookes Publishing Company, Post Office Box 10624, Baltimore, MD 21204. 1985, 427pp.*

The theme of this book is stated in the introduction by the editors: to "offer workers in developmental disabilities and gerontology an opportunity to explore the significant issues that affect the lives of older mentally retarded and developmentally disabled persons". A variety of authors (most of whom are university professors) have contributed twenty six chapters to give a better understanding of the aging process as it applies to persons who have been disabled throughout their lifespans. A variety of perspectives represent the sections of the book: I-Issues in Aging and Disablement, II-Philosophical and Legal Consideration, III-The Older Developmentally Disabled Population, IV-Biological and Clinical Aspects of Aging, V-Service Approaches, VI-Residential Services and VII-Roles and Perspectives.

At some length, the population is defined and current difficulties in the definition are enumerated, e.g., what chronological age represents "old age" for persons with developmental disabilities? The central theme stated by all the authors is that aging developmentally disabled persons represent a growing population, that their need for services is likewise increasing and that present service delivery systems are in need of expansion and alteration if the future needs are to be met. Discussion of needs regarding public policy, approaches to planning administering and delivering services for older developmentally disabled persons follows.

Chapters on the epidemiology, demography and genetics of aging and public policy planning seem excessively long and detailed for the clinically oriented reader. Chapters on such subjects as psychological processes in aging, musculoskeletal aging, nutritional needs, service needs, day activity and residential needs of aging developmentally disabled persons seem more pertinent and interesting. Much of what is presented in these chapters will sound familiar to occupational therapists who have worked with the older and/or developmentally disabled populations.

Although occupational therapy is mentioned briefly with regard to a few issues such as feeding evaluations and residential services, there is a notable absence of occupational therapy in some areas that would seem appropriate, such as day activity programs. Perhaps this is because the book looks to the future and clearly sees a time when most services for this population will be community based. The message seems clear for our profession, if we wish to serve this population, our services need to be available where they are needed: in smaller, community based settings whether they be in residential or in day activity programs.

Stephanie Day, MA, OTR

CHILDREN WITH AUTISM AND OTHER PERVASIVE DISORDERS OF DEVELOPMENT AND BEHAVIOR: THERAPY THROUGH ACTIVITIES. David L. Nelson, PhD, OTR. *Slack, Inc., 6900 Grove Road, Thorofare, NJ 08086; 263 pp, 1984.*

This book offers a unique perspective on treatment programming for autistic children—a comprehensive multidisciplinary approach that is based on fundamental principles of occupational therapy. Nelson's central theme is that concepts from the occupational therapy literature can be put into practice as "activities therapy" by professionals of many disciplines, including special education, psychology, dance therapy, recreation therapy, and so on, to help children with autism and related developmental disorders. Beginning with the premise that participation in purposeful activities is the sine qua non of development, Nelson goes on to present a graphic model of the "whole" child that integrates occupational performance tasks (work, play, and self-care) with underlying component abilities (sensory, motor, perceptual, cognitive, emotional, and interpersonal). This model serves as an organizing framework for discussion of characteristics of autistic children and clinical issues related to evaluation and treatment.

In the introduction to the book, the author states that his intent is to familiarize professionals of all disciplines with the overall needs of autistic children, not to emphasize the importance of a single profession (occupational therapy). His vision of an occupational therapy perspective guiding special services for autistic children is an exciting one, and may lead to more widespread appreciation of the value of this profession. On the other hand, the embedding of occupational therapy concepts within "activities therapy" may further obscure a profession that already lacks visibility. Although Nelson cites numerous occupational therapy authors, he seldom indicates explicitly which of his concepts were derived from this profession. Every occupational therapist will recognize the process of activity analysis and synthesis advocated by Nelson, but other professionals may not realize that this is an elemental principle of occupational therapy.

For occupational therapists, this book will probably be of greatest value to those who are encountering autistic children for the first time. Nelson discusses diagnostic issues, lists appropriate evaluation tools, and directs the reader to additional sources of information. The review of strengths and weaknesses of austistic children is exceptionally thorough and should be useful to novice and experienced therapists alike.

Special attention is given to behavior modification and to sensorimotor or sensory integrative approaches, all of which are viewed as appropriate for inclusion in activities therapy. The coverage of behavioral techniques is strong and is likely to make this book a helpful reference to occupational therapists and other professionals who work in settings that routinely use behavioral methods. In contrast, the chapter on sensorimotor and sensory integrative approaches is superficial; therapists interested in using these approaches will need to seek out more indepth information elsewhere. Nelson is careful to indicate the strengths and limitations of both behavioral and sensorimotor approaches. However, he does not articulate how such different theoretical perspectives can be applied together, nor does he forewarn of the conflicts that can arise between them in practice. For example, in dealing with self-stimulatory behaviors of autistic children, use of a behavioral approach can lead to an entirely different set of therapeutic procedures than use of a sensory integrative one. It is left to the reader to detect and resolve complex issues such as this.

In summary, *Children With Autism* promises to be a useful reference for therapists faced with the perplexing challenge of treating an autistic child. While it offers a broad survey of treatment approaches, its strong behavioral orientation will probably make it most useful for professionals who work in programs that employ behavior modification techniques.

Diane Parham, MA, OTR

STAFF DEVELOPMENT IN MENTAL RETARDATION SER-VICES—A PRACTICAL HANDBOOK. James F. Gardner and Michael S. Chapman. *Paul H. Brookes Publishing Co., P.O. Box 10624, Baltimore, MD 21285-0624; 1985, 319pp, $19.95.*

This book was designed for students and staff providing services to persons with mental retardation. The aim is to provide a review of basic skills, knowledge and values required for successful service delivery. Topics covered include Normalization, Legal Rights, Assessment, Interdisciplinary Team Process, Developing Instructional Strategies, Behavior Observation and Management, Maintaining Safe Environments, Drugs and Medications, Human Sexuality, Working with Stress and Burnout, and Management Responsibilities.

The chapters are designed as interactive learning and orientation packages. Each begins with learning objectives, proceeds to content, includes learning exercises then concludes with a self-appraisal and a simulated experience using a case study. In addition, key points are highlighted, e.g.,

---

OVERPROTECTION PREVENTS PEOPLE
FROM LEARNING

---

and many main ideas are presented in Table format.

The content of the book is current and very relevant for all professionals providing service to mentally retarded persons. It is most appropriate for students and/or inexperienced professionals. The format of the book is very sound educationally, "as research has demonstrated the most effective learning occurs through self-guided experientially based processes."

My one concern with the book is related to scope of content and the emphasis on behavioral modification as the only treatment focus. However this concern does not negate its usefulness as a training tool for students and entry level staff.

Shirley Vulpe, EdD, OTR